CLINICAL SURGERY
MADE EASY®

CLINICAL SURGERY MADE EASY®

R Thirunavukarasu MS

Professor and Head
Department of Surgery
Vinayaka Missions Medical College
Karaikal, Puducherry, India

Formerly
Head
Department of Surgery
Thanjavur Medical College
Thanjavur, Tamil Nadu, India

JAYPEE BROTHERS MEDICAL PUBLISHERS (P) LTD

New Delhi • London • Philadelphia • Panama

Jaypee Brothers Medical Publishers (P) Ltd

Headquarters
Jaypee Brothers Medical Publishers (P) Ltd
4838/24, Ansari Road, Daryaganj
New Delhi 110 002, India
Phone: +91-11-43574357
Fax: +91-11-43574314
Email: jaypee@jaypeebrothers.com

Overseas Offices
J.P. Medical Ltd
83 Victoria Street, London
SW1H 0HW (UK)
Phone: +44-2031708910
Fax: +02-03-0086180
Email: info@jpmedpub.com

Jaypee Medical Inc
The Bourse
111 South Independence Mall East
Suite 835, Philadelphia, PA 19106, USA
Phone: + 267-519-9789
Email: joe.rusko@jaypeebrothers.com

Jaypee Brothers Medical Publishers (P) Ltd
Shorakhute, Kathmandu
Nepal
Phone: +00977-9841528578
Email: jaypee.nepal@gmail.com

Jaypee-Highlights Medical Publishers Inc
City of Knowledge, Bld. 237, Clayton
Panama City, Panama
Phone: + 507-301-0496
Fax: + 507-301-0499
Email: cservice@jphmedical.com

Jaypee Brothers Medical Publishers (P) Ltd
17/1-B Babar Road, Block-B, Shaymali
Mohammadpur, Dhaka-1207
Bangladesh
Mobile: +08801912003485
Email: jaypeedhaka@gmail.com

Website: www.jaypeebrothers.com
Website: www.jaypeedigital.com

Inquiries for bulk sales may be solicited at: jaypee@jaypeebrothers.com

This book has been published in good faith that the contents provided by the author contained herein are original, and is intended for educational purposes only. While every effort is made to ensure accuracy of information, the publisher and the author specifically disclaim any damage, liability, or loss incurred, directly or indirectly, from the use or application of any of the contents of this work. If not specifically stated, all figures and tables are courtesy of the author. Where appropriate, the readers should consult with a specialist or contact the manufacturer of the drug or device.

Clinical Surgery Made Easy®

First Edition: **2013**

ISBN 978-93-5090-406-0
Printed at: S.Narayan & Sons

Dedicated to

*My beloved parents
and
my children*

Preface

This book mainly aims to help the exam-going undergraduates in surgery and gives a comprehensive study of clinical surgery.

The points in various common surgical cases are grouped in different chapters to help the students easily remember and reproduce in the clinical examinations.

This book also contains essential surgical anatomy, terms and signs as a pocket reference. All common topics are synapsed to aid the students for easy revision.

This book aims to help the exam-going final year students for a quick revision.

You are going to pass in the first attempt...

Wishing you best of luck

R Thirunavukarasu

Acknowledgments

My heartfelt thanks to Dr Sandeep, Dr Shankaraman and Dr Sunil, for their assistance in compilation and clinical photographs.

My sincere thanks to Shri Jitendar P Vij (Group Chairman), Mr Ankit Vij (Managing Director) and Mr Tarun Duneja (Director-Publishing) of M/s Jaypee Brothers Medical Publishers (P) Ltd, New Delhi, India, particularly to Mr Jayanandan (Chennai Branch), for the kind help rendered.

Contents

Points in TAO

TAO (THROMBO ANGITIS OBLITERANS)

1. Affects
   i. Young male
   ii. Smoker

2. Involves
   i. Medium
   ii. Small sized vessels

3. Pathology
   i. Thrombosis—progressive obliteration of vessels
   ii. Panarteritis
       Periarterial fibrosis may involve vein + nerve + lymphatics

4. Clinical Features
   i. Claudication → rest pain
   ii. Gangrene of extremities

5. History of
   i. Thrombophlebitis of superficial and deep veins
   ii. Raynaud's phenomenon

6. Other Examinations
   i. CVS for embolic manifestations
   ii. Diabetic status

7. Description of
   i. The gangrenous area
   ii. Peripheral pulse chart

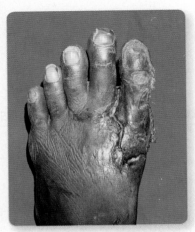

Figure 1.1: TAO—dry gangrene toe

8. Diagnosed by
   i. Blood lipid profile + sugar
   ii. Doppler ultrasonography
   iii. Duplex scanning
   iv. Arteriography
9. Management
   i. Cessation of smoking
   ii. Conservative:
       Vasodilators - doubtful value care of the gangrenous area
   iii. Palliative:
        Amputate the gangrenous area; lumbar sympathectomy for ulcer
   iv. Curative:
       Thromboendarterectomy
       Bye-pass surgery
       Omental graft

· Finding remedy is better than finding fault

10. Gangrene
   i. Dry   Slow progressive arterial (putrefactive necrosis) occlusion with normal venous flow.
   ii. Wet   Simultaneous occlusion of artery + vein sudden arterial occlusion

11. Raynaud's Phenomenon
   W White color of affected area with blanching
   B Blue color due to stagnation of deoxygenated blood.
   C Red color due to oxygentated blood.

PULSE CHART

1.	Dorsalis Pedis	Lateral to extensor hallucis longus tendon at the proximal end of first web space against medial cuneiform bone.
2.	Posterior Tibial	Midway between medial malleolus and tendoachilles, against calcaneum.
3.	Popliteal	Supine position - Knee flexed; felt against tibial condyle Prone position - Knee flexed; felt against femoral condyle.
4.	Femoral Artery	Below mid inguinal point against head of femur with hip joint flexed, abducted and externally rotated.
5.	Radial Pulse	Proximal to the wrist against lower end of radius.

6.	Brachial Pulse	Medial to the biceps tendon against medial humeral condyle.
7.	Axillary	Against humerus head in the axilla.
8.	Subclavian	Supraclavicular fossa in the midclavicular line against first rib.
9.	Common Carotid	At the level of upper border of thyroid cartilage against transvese process of C6 vertebra.
10.	Superficial Temporal	Anterior to the tragus against temporal bone.

Rest Pain: Severe continuous pain in the limb at rest due to severe ischemia (cry of dying nerve).

Claudication Distance: The patient often complains of pain after walking a distance.

Claudication Grades (Boyd):

G1 Pain on walking—pain relieved by continued walking.

G2 Pain on walking—pain worsened, the patient continues to walk.

G3 The pain mostly compels the patient to take rest.

Buerger's Test: Elevation of the ischemic limb causes marked pallor of limb.

(normal limb—no change even on elevation to 90°)

Buerger's Angle: The angle at which sudden pallor develops.

- Abilities not used are abilities wasted
- Many look but only few see

chapter 2

Points in Hernia, Varicose Veins, Peptic Ulcer—Goo, Carcinoma Stomach

HERNIA

Definition: A hernia is defined as protrusion of whole or part of a viscus through the wall that contains it.

Types: *Inguinal*   i. Direct
                      ii. Indirect
            Femoral
            Fatty hernia of linea alba—
            umblical and paraumblical
            Incisional
            Rare—obturator, lumbar, gluteal, spigelion

Inguinal Hernia

Inspection

- Hernial site, size, shape
- Extent into scrotum [complete (or) incomplete]
- Expansile cough impulse

History of

- Chronic cough
- Exposure to STD—gonorrhea—stricture urethra
- Previous surgery for similar complaint

- Appendicectomy by Rutherford Morrison's muscle cutting incision —injury in iliohypogastric nerve— direct hernia

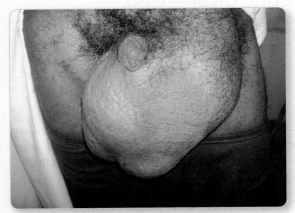

Figure 2.1: Left inguinal hernia

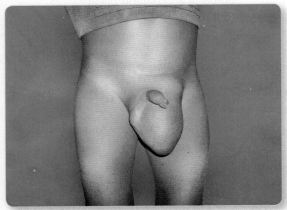

Figure 2.2: Left congenital hernia

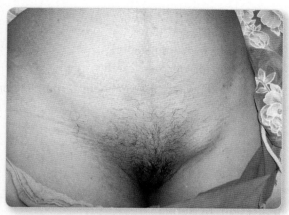

Figure 2.3: Femoral hernia

Palpation
- Describe the hernia—reducibility
- Expansile cough impulse
- Not able to get above the swelling

Tests
- Deep ring occlusion test
- Superficial ring invagination test
- Ziemann's technique of three fingers palpation for deep ring, superficial ring, femoral ring.

Other Examinations
- Other side inguinal region and scrotum
- Penis—meatal stenosis, phimosis, stricture urethra
- Abdomen—malgaigne bulge + PR.

Surgery
- Herniotomy
- Herniorrhaphy
- Hernioplasty

Diagnosis
- Direct (or) indirect
- Compelete (or) incomplete
- Complicated (or) uncomplicated

E.g. : Right sided indirect inguinal hernia, complete and uncomplicated

May Add the Contents
- Enterocele
- Omentocele

Part of Hernial Sac: Mouth, neck, body, fundus

Complications of Hernia
- Irreducibility
- Obstruction
- Strangulation

Getting Above
- To feel the cord structure above the swelling
- Vas deferens felt like fusion thread.
- In pure scrotal swelling this is possible (not in hernia)

Cord Structures
- Vas deferens (round ligament in females)
- Pampiniform plexus of veins
- Artery to testis and vas
- Lymphatics
- Genital branch of genitofemoral nerve

Covered by
- Internal spermatic fascia—from transversalis fascia.
- Cremasteric fascia—from cremastric muscles.

- Disease is the fate of poor, but also punishment of rich—Ivo Andrick

- External spermatic fascia—from external oblique aponeurosis.

Principles of Herniorrhaphy

(Modified Bassini's Procedure)

1. Herniotomy
2. Narrowing of deep ring—lytle's repair
3. Strengthen the posterior wall of inguinal canal by approximating conjoint tendon with inguinal ligament by non-absorbable sutures.
   - Polypropylene (blue colored) non-absorbable synthetic material is used.

Shouldice Procedure : Four layered double breasting repair.

Lichtenstein's -Tension free repair—now commonly done.

Hernioplasty

Indications

- Recurrent hernia
- Weak abdominal wall with large defect
- Elderly patient
  - Prolene (or) dacron mesh is used.

Sliding Hernia

- Hernia with the posterior wall of the sac formed by one of its contents.

Richter's Hernia

- Hernia including part of circumference of the bowel loop.

· Everything has its beauty but not every one sees it

Littre's Hernia

- Meckel's diverticulum is the content.

Pantaloon Hernia

- Combination of direct and indirect

Femoral Hernia

- Herniation through the femoral ring.

Surgery : Aims to obliterate the femoral ring through which the hernia occurs.

Approaches

1. McEvedy   :   Incision above the inguinal ligament (mountain-high) high approach.
2. Lotheissen :   Just above inguinal ligament
3. Lock Wood's : Low incision below Inguinal ligament.

VARICOSE VEINS

Dilated, tortuous, distended visible veins

1. **Patient comes for**
   - Cosmetic problem
   - Pain
   - Ulceration

2. **History of**
   - Occupation
   - Family history
   - Following pregnancy

3. **Inspection**
   - Describe the vein
   - Ulcer
   - Blow outs

4. **Palpation**
   - Fegan's method to mark blow outs
   - Schwartz tapping to know a single column of blood
   - Deep vein status ... Homan's and Moses' tests

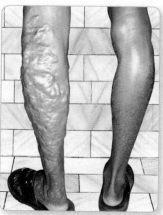

Figure 2.4: Varicose veins

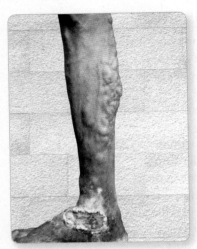

Figure 2.5: Varicose veins with ulcer

Clinical Tests

1. Trendelenburg's test
2. Multiple tourniquet test
3. Modified Perthe's test

Investigation

- Doppler and duplex scan
- Venography
- Ultrasound abodmen.

Treatment

1. Conservative
2. Sclero therapy—injection of sclerosant solution 5% phenol in gingelly oil.
3. Surgery
   - *Trendelenburg's operation*—ligation of constant tributaries of LSV Flush ligation of saphenofemoral junction

- *Cockett and Dodd subfascial* ligation of perforators
- Segmental removal
- **SEPS**—subfascial endoscopic perforator surgery
- *Linton's operation:* Excusion of ulcer with deep fascia + Split skin crafting.

Constant Tributaries of Long Saphenous Vein

1. Superficial circumflex iliac
2. Superficial epigastric
3. Superficial external pudental

Deep pudental—inconstant tributary

Complications

1. Lipodermosclerosis
2. Venous ulcer
3. Equinus deformity
4. Rupture of vein
5. Malignant transformation of ulcer—Marjolin's ulcer

PEPTIC ULCER—GOO

Gastric Outlet Obstruction Due to Cicastrized Duodenal Ulcer

Peptic Ulcer is Due to

- Imbalance between acid secreting mechanism and mucoprotective mechanism.
  1. Gastric ulcer
  2. Duodenal ulcer
  3. Ectopic gastric mucosal ulcer.
     - Jejunum, Meckel's diverticulum etc.

• Trust your hopes, not your fears

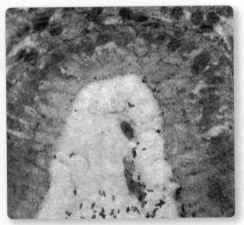

Figure 2.6: *Helicobacter pylori*

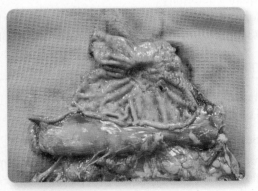

Figure 2.7: Carcinoma stomach—resected specimen

Acid Secretion

1. Cephalic phase
2. Gastric phase
3. Intestinal phase

Factors

1. Neurocrine - Acetylcholine
2. Paracrine - Histamine
3. Endocrine - Gastrin

History of previous episodes of abdominal pain and drug relief.

Family History

General Examination : Watch for signs of dehydration—shrunken eyes, indrawn cheek, dry tongue, loss of skin turgescence.

Inspection of abdomen

1. VGP
2. Dehydration signs.

Palpation

- Succussion splash
- Ausculto percussion to elicit dilated stomach. Greater curvature of stomach is marked.
- Search for any lump in the epigastrium and right hypochondrium. (A case of carcinoma stomach—antral growth).

Investigations

- Fibreoptic endoscopy
- Ultrasonography for other cause of dyspepsia—gallstone
- Barium meal series
  a. Deformed duodenal cap
  b. Delayed emptying
  c. Dilated stomach

Complications of Peptic Ulcer Disease

1. Cicatrisation and scarring
2. Bleeding
3. Perforation

In case of *GOO* as patient is already with the complications of the disease, there is no role for medical treatment such as H_2 receptors antagonists etc.

Prepare the Patient for Surgery

1. Correct the dehydration
2. Correct the electrolyte imbalance
3. Gastric lavage with saline, to reduce the edema and to regain the tone of stomach (receptive relaxation and tonic contraction).

Surgery : PGJ with truncal vagotomy

PVRING—Post, vertical, retrocolic, isoperistaltic, no loop, no tension, gastrojejunostomy

Vagotomy : (Dragstedt)

- Truncal
- Selective
- Highly selective

Vagus : X Cranial Nerve Bilateral

In abdomen, (L) become anterior (R) become posterior (LARP)

Branches of Vagus

Anterior Vagus
- Hepatic
- Branches to acid secreting area
- Nerve of Laterjet—Innervating antrum

· The difference between ordinary and extraordinary is that little extra

Posterior Vagus
- Celiac
- Branches to acid secreting area
- Nerve of Laterjet—Innervating antrum

Medical Treatment for Peptic Ulcer

- Antacids
- H_2 antagonist
- Proton pump inhibitor
- Mucoprotective agents
- Anti *H. pylori* regime:

  Proton Pump Inhibitors + Antibiotics—Clarithromycin or Amoxycillin and Metronidazole for 1 to 2 weeks

Types of Gastric Ulcer

Type I   Ulcer in the junction of acid producing and gastrin secreting cells in the lesser curvature.

Type II   Duodenal ulcer with stasis ulcer in stomach

Type III   Pre-pyloric ulcer.

Type IV   Ulcer in the proximal stomach or cardia.

CARCINOMA STOMACH

- Lump in the epigastrium and right hypochondrium
- Antral growth—VGP ++

Predisposing Factors

1. Smoking and spirit
2. Atrophic gastritis
3. Pernicious anemia
4. Polyp
5. Post-gastric surgery stump

• It takes five years to learn when to operate and twenty years to learn when not to

6. *Helicobacter pylori* infection
7. Dietary factors : Smoked food, Increased salt, nitrate
8. Blood group 'A'

Clinical Signs of Inoperability

1. Secondaries in liver
2. Virchow's node
3. Free fluid in the peritoneal cavity
4. Krukenberg's tumors of ovary
5. Blumer's shelf—deposits in the rectovesical area, rectouterine pouch—made out by PR
6. Sister Joseph's nodule in umbilicus.

Palliative Procedures

1. AGJ
2. Devine's exclusion procedure
3. Feeding gastrostomy/Jejunostomy

Operable Cases

- Total radical gastrectomy with [esophagojejunostomy Roux-en-y]
- Subtotal radical gastrectomy.

Points in Hydrocele

HYDROCELE

Definitive
Increased accumulation of fluid between the two layers of tunica vaginalis

Causes
1. Increased secretion
2. Decreased absorption
3. Blockade of lymphatic drainage
4. Persistence of communication to peritoneal cavity by processus vaginalis.

Clinical Examination
1. Fluctuant soft swelling—elicit fluctuation in two opposite directions.
2. Transillumination + ve if content of the sac is a clear fluid and containing wall must be thin to allow light rays to penetrate through them.
3. Able to get above the swelling—purely scrotal.
4. Palpate the testis—not palpable in primary hydrocele.

Complications
1. Hematocele
2. Pyocele
3. Relative impotency
4. Herniation of hydrocele sac
5. Rupture

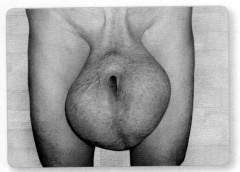

Figure 3.1: Bilateral hydrocele

Surgery

1. Bilateral eversion of sac (Andrew's)
2. Partial excison and eversion of sac (Jaboulay's)
3. Total excision of sac.
4. Lord's plication (for small, thin walled sac)
5. Congenital hydrocele is treated by herniotomy

Principle of Surgery

1. Exposing the secreting surface to larger area to facilitate resorption.
2. As time goes, secreting epithlium loses its secreting capacity.

Types

Etiopathological

I   Acquired

–   Primary—idiopathic

- What is beautiful is not always good; but what is good is always beautiful

- Secondary
    1. Filariasis
    2. TB epididymitis
    3. Testicular tumor
    4. Syphilitic orchitis

II Developmental
1. Congential
2. Infantile
3. Funicular
4. Encysted hydrocele of the cord

Difference

Primary	Secondary
1. Large, tense	Small and lax
2. Testis not palpable	Testis palpable
3 No other abnormality	Secondary causes like filariasis, tumor, TB epididymitis, made out
4. Transudate	Exudate

- People can be divided into three types; those who make things happen, those who watch things happen and those who wonder what is happening

Points in Thyroid, Obstructive Jaundice, Carcinoma Breast and Portal Hypertension

THYROID

Presentations

1. Primary hyperthyroidism with diffuse goiter
2. Secondary hyperthyroidism with multinodular goiter
3. Solitary nodule thyroid
4. Carcinoma thyroid
5. Colloid goiter
6. MNG—non-toxic

Inspection

1. Describe the swelling and end the statement saying it moves with deglutition.
2. Whether you are able to see the lower border on deglutition.
3. Size and extent of swelling in relation to upper border of thyroid cartilage above and suprasternal notch below, laterally sternocleidomastoid muscle.
4. Presence of enlarged veins on the anterior surface.
5. Position of trachea.

- A surgeon should have a heart of a lion, eyes of a hawk and hands of a women

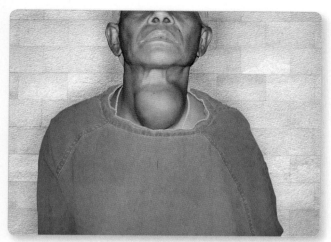

Figure 4.1: Colloid goiter

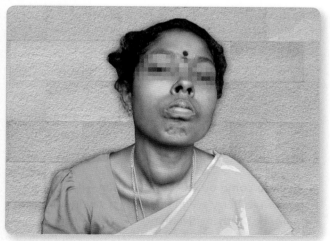

Figure 4.2: Multinodular goiter

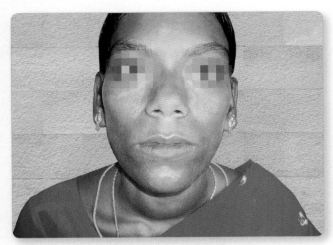

Figure 4.3: Toxic Thyroid

Palpation

1. Palpate the swelling size, shape, consistency, surface, border, etc.
2. Assess the plane of the swelling
   - Skin pinchable
   - Deep to investing layer of deep fascia
   - Deep to infrahyoid strap muscles—sternothyroid, sternohyoid and thyrohyoid [less prominent on contraction of the muscle]
3. Position of trachea
4. Palpate common carotid pulsation—if absent, it is known as Berry's Sign Positive (in carcinoma due to carotid sheath involvement).
5. Regional lymph node—movement on deglutition due to attachment to the larynx and trachea by Berry's ligament.

Berry's Ligaments: One in each side, condensation of the posterior layer of pretracheal fascia enclosing thyroid attached to the cricoid cartilage and thyroid cartilage below the oblique line.

Thrill is palpated in the superior pole. Superior thyroid artery is the main feeding artcry. Superficially palpable in toxic thyroid due to increased vascular supply.

Arterial Supply to the Thyroid

1. Superior thyroid artery—branch of external carotid artery.
2. Inferior thyroid artery—branch of thyrocervical trunk.
3. Arteria thyroid ima—branch of arch of aorta.
4. Unnamed branches from tracheal and
5. Esophageal vessels.

Structures That Moves on Deglutition

1. Thyroid
2. Thyroglossal cyst (also moves on protrusion of tongue)
3. Sub-hyoid bursa
4. Pre-tracheal lymph nodes
5. Pre-laryngeal lympth nodes

D/D Solitary Nodule Thyroid

1. Dominant nodule MNG
2. Adenoma
3. Carcinoma
4. Thyroid cyst
5. Localized Hashimoto's disease

• Importance of passing urine is realized only when you cannot pass the urine

Primary Thyrotoxicosis	**Secondary**
(Graves' disease)	
1. Age (young women)	Middle age
2. Diffuse swelling	Nodular
3. Toxicity appears along with swelling or even present before the appearance of the swelling	Swelling first appears next symptoms
4. Eye sign + ve	Eye sign −ve
5. CNS involvement more	CVS involvement more

Tertiary Toxicity : Term describing toxicity in solitary nodule thyroid.

Investigation

1. **FNAC:** Draw back: It can not differentiate follicular carcinoma from follicular adenoma. It is only the study of the cells, the follicular malignancy involves pericapsular, vascular invasions which cannot be made out by FNAC. FNAB help to distinguish.

2. Thyroid profile: Total T_4

   Free T_3

   TSH

3. Isotope studying in solitary nodule

   Cold nodule   -   Mostly malignancy

   Warm   -   Euthyroid

   Hot nodule   -   Hyperthyroid

   Mainly done in cases of toxicity in association with Nodularity.

4. AMA—antimicrosomal antibody

5. Ultrasound if cystic swelling

• Anger is a short madness which often causes life-long tragedy
• You are born alone, die alone and meet the examiners alone

6. X-ray neck to know the tracheal position, calcification
7. Sleeping pulse chart in a case of thyroid toxicity.
8. ENT examination—for position of the vocal cords.
9. X-ray chest, ECG—rhythm disturbance
10. Blood-Grouping and typing—reserve blood/urea, sugar, creatinine, etc.

Diagnosis : Say whether it is toxic and whether it is malignant.

E.g.: Non-toxic, non malignant MNG

Surgical Procedures : For toxic thyroid—bring the patient to euthyroid level prior to surgery

1. Subtotal thyroidectomy (aggressive)—(for toxic thyroid)—removal of enlarged thyroid even upto 7/8th of enlargement (should leave 1/3rd of size of normal gland—corresponding to the thumb size of patient)
2. Adequate subtotal thyroidectomy—for cosmetic reason in colloid goiter and non-toxic goiter.
3. Hemi thyroidectomy—removal of one lobe and isthmus
4. Near total thyroidectomy—removal of gland leaving a small part of thyroid in the tracheoesophageal groove.
5. Total thyroidectomy—removal of entire thyroid gland.

Complications of Thyroid Surgery

During Surgery :

1. Injury to the vessels—carotid, jugular
2. Injury to the nerves—RLN, SLN
3. Injury to the oesophagus
4. Injury to the trachea
5. Parathyroid glands injury

Postoperative :

1. Hemorrhage
   - Primary
   - Reactionary—within 24 hours
   - Secondary—7 to 10 days

   The occurrence of clot in the closed space causes respiratory distress. Immediately the wound must be opened up and clot evacuated from the wound. Then proceed with management in the theatre.

2. Thyroid storm (crisis)
   - It is an acute exacerbation of hyperthyroidism
   - It occurs in a thyrotoxic patient inadequately prepared for thyroidectomy

3. Tetany—due to parathyroid injury—hypocalcemia

4. Tracheal obstruction

5. Hypothyroidism

Eye Signs in Thyrotoxicosis

1. Stellwag's sign—starring look
2. Von Graefe's sign—lid lag
3. Joffroy's sign—absenc of wrinkle
4. Dairymple's sign—lid retraction
5. Moebius sign—not able to converge medially

OBSTRUCTIVE JAUNDICE [SURGICAL JAUNDICE]

1. Obstructive Jaundice is defined as jaundice due to obstruction to the excretion of bile.
2. Surgical Jaundice refers to jaundice due to extrehepatic obstruction that can be treated surgically.

Causes

1. Intrahepatic
   - Cholestatic stage of infective hepatitis
   - Drug induced cholestasis

2. Extrahepatic
   1. Gallstones—impacted
   2. Carcinoma head of the pancreas
   3. Periampullary carcinoma
   4. CBD—Stricture + Stenosis
   5. Node in the porta hepatis

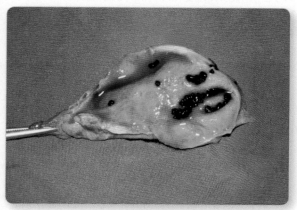

Figure 4.4: Gall stones

- Surgery is not just cutting, but it is an art; not only an art but also a merciful art

Clinical Features
- Progressive or intermittenet jaundice
- High colored urine
- Clay colored stool
- Pruritis.

History of
1. History of attack of pain with appearance of jaundice
2. History of blood transfusion
3. Any previous surgery: [Anesthetic agents may produce jaundice].

Investigations
1. Urine [bile salts + ve, bile pigments + ve, urobilinogen – ve]
2. Serum bilirubin [conjugated increased]
3. Serum alkaline phosphatase increased
4. Prothrombin time—prolonged
5. Ultrasound the standard investigation
   ERCP—Therapeutic as well as diagnostic lower CBD visualization
   PTC—Invasive, useful in high obstruction
   MRCP—Recent non-invasive investigation

Tips for Palpation
- Palpate for GB
  If enlarged, cause is usually carcinoma head of pancreas or periampullary carcinoma.
  (Remember Courvoisier`s law: In obstructive jaundice, if GB is enlarged it is not due to Gallstones.).

If GB is not Palpable
- Examine for any primary malignant focus.
  E.g. carcinoma stomach, node in the porta hepatis will be the cause for obstructive jaundice.
- Look for previous surgical scars—injury to biliary system

• It is when the fish opens his mouth that he gets caught

Surgery in Jaundiced Patients: Problems
1. **Infected bile under pressure**
    - Prophylactic antibiotics
    - Preoperative drainage
        - Endoscopic stenting or Sphincterotomy
2. **Risk of renal failure: Hepato renal syndrome**
    - Adequate hydration
    - Osmotic diuresis during surgery (mannitol)
    - Catheterization to monitor output
3. **Impaired hepatic detoxification**
    - Antibiotics to minimise endogenous endotoxins—oral neomycin
    - Avoid drugs excreted by liver
4. **Impaired protein synthesis**
    - Check clotting
    - Injection vit. K. One week prior

Whipple's Procedure : Definitive surgery for carcinoma head of pancreas and periampullary carcinoma. Also known as pancreatico- duodenectomy
1. Cholecystectomy
2. Truncal vagotomy and antrectomy
3. Removal of head of pancreas and duodenum

Triple anastomosis
1. Pancreatojejunostomy
2. Choledochojejunostomy
3. GJ

Inoperable Carcinoma Head of Pancreas

Do triple anastomosis palliatively
- GB to jejunum
    - the obstruction to bile flow is relieved

- Stomach to jejunum
  - prophylactive
- Jejunum to jejunum
  - the biliary secretion is prevented from going to stomach.

Gallstones

90%   Radiolucent

10%   Radiopaque

1. Mixed stones (75–90%): Combination of bile pigments, calcium salts and cholesterol—multiple
2. Cholesterol stones (10%)—large, solitary
3. Pigment stones: Calcium bilirubinate—multiple, black
4. Calcium carbonate stones—rare, grey colored

R_x : Cholecystectomy

Indications for Exploration of CBD

1. H/O Jaundice / Cholangitis
2. Diameter of C.B.D $\geq$1 cm
3. Palpable and US evidence of stone in the C.B.D.
4. Multiple stone and biliary mud
5. Elevated alkaline phosphatase.

CARCINOMA BREAST

History

1. H/O Lump

   Origin, duration + progress

   ± Pain (usually painless)

2. Discharge from nipple
   - Spontaneous
   - Bloody discharge D/D Duct papilloma, Carcinoma Breast

3. Any H/O Nipple retraction—recent

4. Loss of appetite + weight

Past H/O

1. Any previous breast surgery

   (Benign lump with pathological report of atypical epithelial hyperplasia needs close follow-up)

2. Use of oral contraceptive pills.

3. Hormone replacement therapy in postmenopausal woman.

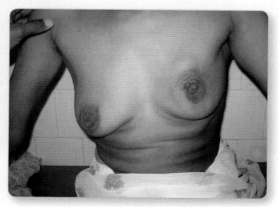

Figure 4.5: Carcinoma breast left

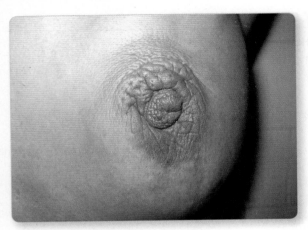

Figure 4.6: Carcinoma breast

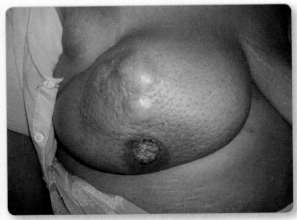

Figure 4.7: Carcinoma breast

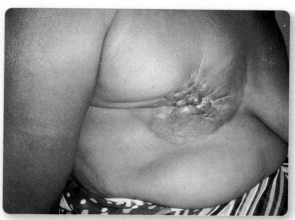

Figure 4.8: Recurrent carcinoma breast

Menstrual, Marital + Lactational History

1. Menarche-age
2. Marriage-age
3. Age of 1st pregnancy
4. Lactation
5. Menopause
- Early menarche + late menopause with prolonged menstrual cycles predispose to carcinoma breast.
- Lactation is believed to give some protection.
- If first child is born after 30 years, there is increased chances of malignancy.
- Unmarried women and nulliparity are also precipitating factors.

Family H/O : Whether any first degree relatives affected by carcinoma breast (mother, sister and daughter).

Personal H/O : High fat + protein diet + higher socioeconomic status —increased chances of carcinoma breast.

On Examination : Patient stripped upto waist :

1. Arms by the side
2. Arms raised above the head
3. Hands on hip-relaxed + pressed
4. Patient leaning forwards
   - Compare both breasts—size, shape, level of nipple + areola.
   - Nipple—depressed, destroyed, displaced, deviated or duplicated.
   - If lump is visible, describe the size, shape, extent, quadrant occupied, skin.

Cutaneous Manifestations of Carcinoma Breast

1. Dimpling or Tethering involvement of ligament of Cooper.
2. Infiltration
3. Peau de' orange (orange peel appearance)
   — Subcuticular lymphoedema with pitting at the sites of hair follicles.
4. Cancer—encuirasse—armor chest
5. Ulceration
6. Paget's disease of nipple with excoriation

Palpation

1. Site, size, shape, surface, edges and consistency carcinoma breast lump is usually—painless, dominant, discrete, dense, different from rest of breast tissue, hard in consistency with irregular margin.

• Man can not discover new oceans unless he has courage to lose sight of the shore

2. Assess the fixity to skin, to the pectoral fascia, muscle and to chest wall.
3. Look for any other lump in all quadrants.
4. Examine axillary lymph nodes, size of the node, consistency, mobility and the group it belongs to
    – pectoral group—anterior
    – brachial—lateral
    – central
    – posterior
    – apical
5. Never forget to palpate the other breast, axilla, supraclavicular area.

Examination Abdomen

1. Liver enlargement
2. Presence of free fluid
3. In pre-menopausal women for any ovarian lump (Krukenberg tumor)
4. PR—for evidence of 'Blummer Shelf'—malignant deposit in the pouch of Douglas.

Respiratory System: For pleural effusion, metastatic deposits—in case of bone pain, examine region of pain particularly:

1. Spine,
2. Ribs,
3. Upper end of femur and humerus.

Diagnosis Must Be Told With Involved Area, Clinical Staging + TNM Status

E.g.:Carcinoma right breast upper and outer quadrant
    stage-I
    T_1 N_0 M_0

Management:
- Investigation
  +
- Treatment

Investigation

1. To confirm the clinically made diagnosis
2. To find the extent of spread of disease
3. To assess the patient for anesthesia + Surgery
   - FNAC
   - If inconclusive, Trucut Biopsy
   - Mammography
   - X-ray chest

In Advanced Cases
- LFT
- Serum alkaline phosphatase
- Urinary carcinoma and hydroxyproline
- X-ray of the site of symptoms
- Isotope scintigraphy of bones
- CT scan

Treatment

- Early carcinoma—operable carcioma
  Clinical Stage I + II (T_1 - T_2 - T_3 - N_0 - N_1 - M_0)
- Modified radical mastectomy specimen is sent for histopathological examination in formalin 10%; part of it packed with ice and sent for estrogen receptor status study within 30 minutes
- If node is positive for malignancy, adjuvant chemotherapy is given despite the receptor status
- If node is negative but ER + ve, Tamoxifen is given.

Lymph Node Clearance of Axilla

Level - I Lateral to pectoralis minor (low)
     II Deep to pectoralis minor (middle)
    III Medial to pectoralis minor (high)

Advanced Carcinoma

Inoperable carcinoma—clinical Stage III + IV (T_3 - T_4 - N_2, M_1), the treatment is only palliative

- Radiotherapy to the breast + axilla
- Chemotherapy to be followed
- Tamoxifen is also given

If ulceration of the breast is present, palliative total mastectomy done followed by chemotherapy.

Chemotherapy : CMF Regime

1. Cyclophosphamide 100/mg/m^2 orally or daily for 14 days. IV 600 mg/m^2 on day 1+ 8
2. Methotrexate 40 mg / m^2—IV, day 1+ 8
3. 5 - Fluorouracil 600 mg/m^2—IV, day 1 + 8

Cycle repeated every 4 weeks

For a period of 6 months

Before next administration of hemotherapy look for

- WBC count - (should not be less than 4000 / Cu.mm)
- Platelet count > 1,00,000, Hb > 8 gms.
- Adriamycin is replacing methotrexate now a days.

Side Effect of CMF Regime

1. Myelosuppression bone marrow function to be monitored
2. Immunosuppression
   - Control infection
3. Carcinogenesis
   - Cyclophosphamide induces leukemia and bladder Carcinoma.

Tamoxifen

- Dosage of 10–20 mg BD
- Anti-estrogen—act by competitive blocking
- Side effects :   Hot flushes
                    Uterine bleed
                    Thrombophlebitis
                    Rash
- For a period of 4 to 5 years.
- Contra : Past H/O Thromboembolism
  Abnormal uterine bleeding.

PORTAL HYPERTENSION
(RARELY KEPT AS A LONG CASE)

Clinical Presentations

1. Hepatosplenomegaly with history of hematemesis and melena
2. Splenomegaly with history of hematemesis
3. Only splenomegaly—no history of hematemesis
4. History of hematemesis only—spleen shrunken due to recent bleed and liver not palpable. One and two type of presentation will be kept in the examination.

History

1. History of presenting complaints
   - Lump, etc.
2. History of hematemesis
   - Color
   - Quantity and episodes
   - Loss of consciousness during an episode of hematemesis is important to know whether disease is compensated or decompensated.
3. Regarding D/D for hematemesis
   - Peptic ulcer
   - Intake of ulcerogenic drugs
   - NSAID, aspirin, steroids, anti-TB drugs, etc.
4. Regarding D/D Splenomegaly
   - History of fever with chills for parasitic disease
   - History of bleeding gums, bone pain, lymphadenopathy for Reticuloendothelial disease
5. History of jaundice
6. History of alcoholism

Past History of : Treatment Taken

1. Transfusion
2. Diuretics
3. Salt restriction
4. History of upper GI endoscopy
5. Treatment for varices

General Examination

1. Sign of dehydration, anemia
2. Nutritional status
3. Evidence for liver failure
   - Palmar erythema
   - Spider naevi
   - Gynecomastia
   - Testicular atrophy
   - Loss of axillary and pubic hair
   - Icterus
   - Ascites
   - Ecchymotic patches over the body due to coagulation defects
   - Fetor hepaticus.

Abdomen

- **Look for hepatomegaly and splenomegaly.**
- **Spleen**
  - Lump in left hypochondrium, moves with respiration
  - Presence of splenic notch
  - Enlargement towards RIF
  - Not able to insinuate fingers between costal margin and lump.
  - Huge spleen may be bimanually palpable but not ballotable.

- **Liver**
    - Right hypochondrium and epigastrium
    - Enlarging downwards-edge felt
    - Insinuation of fingers between lump and costal margin not possible
    - Not bimanually palpable or ballotable
    - Dullness continues with liver dullness
- **Look for evidence of free fluid**
    - Less than 200 CC—puddle sign
    Percussion around umbilicus patient on knee chest position.
    - More than 500 CC—shifting dullness
    - More than 1 litre—fluid thrill
    - Horseshoe dullness

Auscultation : Venous hum over umbilicus
Cruveilhier-Baumgarten syndrome.

Systemic Examination

CVS—for systolic soft hemic murmur
RS—for pleural effusion.

Diagnosis : Congestive splenomegaly due to portal hypertension secondary to cirrhosis - (commonly).

Investigations

1. US abdomen
    - To know the state of liver and spleen
    - Presence of free fluid
    - Condition of the portal vein (patent or obstructed), splenic vein and collaterals.
2. Upper GI endoscopy
    - For grading the varices
    - To rule out peptic ulcer.

3. Liver function tests and complete hemogram
4. IV Urography—to evaluate left renal function (for lienorenal shunt)
5. Splenoportography
   - Done in patients considered for surgery (not done in child's B and C)
   - To know splenic pulp pressure
   - Condition of splenic vein and portal vein
   - Intrahepatic pattern
   - Collaterals—esophagus and gastric varices.
6. Liver biopsy—liver scan—to exclude hepatomas
7. Severity of liver disease is graded accordingy to

Child's Classification		*Points*	
Tip : **ABCDE**	1	2	3
1. Serum **A**lbumin (g/100 mL)	>3.5	3–3.5	<3
2. Serum **B**ilurubin (mg/100 mL)	<2	2–3	>3
3. **C**lotting Status Prothrombin time (seconds prolonged)	<2	3–5	>5
4. **D**istension Ascites	None	Mild/ moderate	Severe
5. **E**ncephalopathy	None	Minim	Moderate /severe

A = 5–7 Points
B = 8–9 Points
C = 10–15 Points

Indication for Elective Surgery in PHT

1. Bleeding esophageal varices—once they have bled, they will bleed again
   (Absolute Indication)
2. Hypersplenism and Ascites—relative indication

Ideal Patient for Shunt Operation

1. Under 45 years.
2. Category A or B with inactive liver disease
3. Should look well and feel well.

Shunt Procedures

1. Portocaval
2. Lienorenal
3. Mesocaval
4. Selective Decompression Warren's Operation : Distal Lienorenal Shunt without Splenectomy

Non Surgical Approach

1. Injection sclerotherapy of esophageal varices
   - Cyanoacrylate glue injection or banding—via Endoscope
2. Percutaneous transhepatic embolisation
3. Propranolol for prevention of recurrent hemorrhage.

Emergency Treatment of Bleeding Varices

1. Conservative approach:
   - Blood replacement
   - Intravenous (IV) Vasopressin 20 units in 200 ml of 5% dextrose given in 20 minutes.
   - Somatostatin IV bolus of 250 ug followed by continuous IV infusion of 7.5 ug/minute. Octereotide now used.

- Sengstaken-Blakemore balloon tamponade for 24–48 hours
- Injection vitamin K
- Prehepatic coma prevention
  - Oral non-absorbable antibiotic
  - Colonic washout
  - Lactulose
  - Restriction of proteins
- Injection of 5 mL of 5% enthanolamine oleate using rigid endoscope followed by tamponade.
- Rubber banding for esophageal varices
- Glue injection for fundal varices

Direct Surgery to Varices

- Transthoracic esophageal ligation of varices— (Boeremia - Crile Operation)
- Transthoracic esophagus transection with variceal ligation— (Milnes Walker)
- Transabdominal esophagogastric transection and reunion (Tanner's)
- Subcardiac portoazygos disconnection
- Sugiura procedure, i.e. combined devascularization (Upper stomach, lower esophagus and GE junction transected and reunited)

Recent Advance

- TIPSS (Transjugular Intrahepatic Porto Systemic Shunt)
- Transposition of Palmaz Balloon Expandable Stent between hepatic vein and intrahepatic branches of portal vein via right internal jugular vein.
  - Normal portal venous pressure: 7–8 mm Hg.
  - More than 10 mm Hg → PHT.

- Portal vein is formed by superior mesenteric and splenic veins—no valve.
- PHT opens up extrahepatic portosystemic anastomotic channels. C become engorged and dilated at the junction of esophagus and fundus of the stomach, in retro peritoneal and periumblical collaterals, in anastamotic veins in anorectal regions.
- Progressive enlargement of spleen occurs from vascular engorgement and associated hypertrophy.
- Hemotological consequences are anemia, thrombocytopenia and Leucopenia.
- Ascites due to increased formation of hepatic and splanchnic lymph.
  - Hypoalbuminemia
  - Salt and H_2O retention
  - Increased Aldosterone and ADH levels also contribute.

Examination of Abdominal Lump

LUMP ABDOMEN

Essentials

1. You have to describe the lump in relation to the anatomical regions.
2. You assess the plane of the lump
   a. Whether arising from parietal wall or intra-abdominal.
   b. If intra-abdominal, then find out whether it is intraperitoneal or retroperitoneal
3. With the available history and other clinical evidences, D/D to be made in the order of common occurrence.
4. The Case Sheet must be complete with the list of necessary investigations and management.

History

- C/O Pain or lump in the abdomen
- Site
- Pain
  - Type—continuous, intermittent, colicky, burning, gripping
  - Severity—mild, moderate or severe
  - Progress—progressive or stationary
  - Radiation
  - Relieving factors
  - Aggravating factors

- H/O Vomiting
  - Character
  - Frequency
  - Relation to ingestion of food
- H/O Hemetemesis
- H/O Melena
- H/O Loss of appetite
- H/O Fever
- H/O Loss of weight
- H/O Genitourinary and bowel habits
- Family H/O—similar illness
- Personal H/O—diet, alcohol and smoking
- Menstrual history

Regions of Abdomen

1. Two vertical lines are drawn from midinguinal point towards mid clavicular line.
2. Two horizontal lines are drawn
   - Transpyloric plane: Midway between xiphisternum and umbilicus—lower border of L_1 vertebra.
   - Transtubercular plane: Connecting the tubercles of iliac crest on each side—upper border of L_5 vertebra.

Nine Regions

1. Right hypochondrium
2. Epigastrium
3. Left hypochondrium
4. Umbilical
5. Right lumbar
6. Left lumbar
7. Right iliac fossa

- A drop of ink may make a million think

8. Hypogastrium
9. Left iliac fossa
   - Examine the inguinal and scrotal region
   - Examine the left supraclavicular area for presence of Virchow's node—(in between the two heads of sternomastoid)

Inspection of Abdomen

1. Shape of abdomen
   - Scaphoid
   - Flat
   - Distended
2. Presence of any visible lump
   - Describe the regions occupied
   - Whether the lump moves with respiration or not
   - Whether it becomes less prominent on head raising test or leg raising test if situated in the middle (to distinguish the lump whether it is arising from parietal wall or intra-abdominal).

   In cases of lump in lateral areas, patient is asked to do Valsalva's maneuvre. Then see whether lump becomes less prominent or more prominent.

   Intra-abdominal lump will become less prominent.
3. Position and description of umbilicus
   - Normally situated midway between xiphisternum and pubic symphysis
   - Tanyol's sign—downward displacement of umbilicus due to ascites
   - Umbilicus may be displaced upwards by swelling from pelvis
   - Swelling from one side of abdomen may push umbilicus to the opposite side

- Normally inverted and slightly retracted
- Everted in ascites
- Tucked in obesity
- Sister Joseph's nodule (malignant deposits in visceral carcinoma).
4. Fullness of flanks, renal angle
5. Movement
   - Respiratory—whether all regions move equally with respiration.
   - pulsatile
     - epigastric pulsations may be seen in thin person.
     - midline lump in front of aorta.
   - Peristalsis
     1. Visible gastric peristalsis (VGP)—from left costal margin to right.
     2. Visible colonic peristalsis (VCP)—from right to left costal margin.
     3. Visible intestinal peristalsis (VIP) seen in acute abdomen like intestinal obstruction—step ladder pattern

Inspection

1. Shape
2. Position of umbilicus
3. Abdominal wall—scars, sinuses, dilated veins
4. Loin, groin, renal angle and spine
5. Movements—visible peristalsis, respiratory, pulsation.
6. Description of lump.

General Examination

- Build, nutrition
- Anemia, jaundice
- Clubbing, peripheral edema

- Generalized lymphadenopathy
- Signs of dehydration.

Palpation

1. Temperature
2. Tenderness
3. Confirm the inspectory findings about the lumps, size, shape and surface.
4. Margins—ill defined—Inflammatory or traumatic and well defined—Neoplasm

   Upper border can not be made out—extends under costal margin. Lower border could not be felt (extend into pelvis)
5. Consistency—soft, cystic, firm, hard, uniform or variable.
6. Whether it is parietal or intra-abdominal lump by palpation also.
7. Movement of the lump with respiration swelling in contact with under surface of diaphragm more cephalo caudal with respiration liver-spleen, G.B, stomach, kidney.
   - Mobility in different directions and intrinsic mobility.
   - Ballotement—Renal swelling.
8. Palpate for organomegaly—liver, spleen, kidney.

   To determine the relationship of the lump to them.
   - For presence of liver metastasis.
9. Assess the plane of the lump putting the patient in knee chest position.
   - lump—falls forwards or better felt > intraperitoneal
   - lump—not falling > retroperitoneal.

Percussion

Dull note over solid masses and fluid

1. Liver
2. Spleen
3. Kidney—band of resonance due to transverse colon may be present in dull percussion area.
    - Shifting dullness in the presence of free fluids.
    - Impaired dullness over lump arising out of hollow organs—stomach, intestine, colon, etc.

Ausculation

- Auscultopercussion ⎫
- Succussion splash   ⎬ In case of GOO
                                      ⎭
- Kenawy's sign—venous hum below xiphistemum —PHT.

PR and PV must be done, D/D for intra-abodminal lump.

Right Hypochondrium

Solid

- Liver secondaries, hepatoma
- Carcinoma gall bladder
- Hypernephroma of upper pole of right kidney

Cystic

- Palpable G.B.
- Hydatid cyst
- Hydronephrosis of upper pole of right kidney
- Liver abscess.

Epigastrium

Solid

- Carcinoma stomach
- Liver—hepatoma, secondaries

- Carcinoma colon
- Para-aortic nodes.

Cystic

- Liver abscess
- Hydatid cyst
- Pseudo cyst of pancreas
- Perigastric abscess

Left Hypochondrium

- Enlarged spleen
- Left renal mass
- Left sided colonic mass

Hypogastrium

- Bladder mass
- Uterine mass
- Ovarian mass

Lumbar

Solid

- Carcinoma ascending colon
- Renal carcinoma
- Retroperitoneal tumors

Cystic

- Hydronephrosis
- Polycystic kidney
- Retroperitoneal cyst, pedunculated ovarian cyst.

Umbilical

Solid

- Lymphoma
- Lymphoma/sarcoma of intestine

Cystic
- Omental cyst
- Mesentric cyst.

Right Iliac Fossa (RIF)
- Appendicular lump
- Ilecaecal TB
- Carcinoma cecum / ascending colon
- External iliac lymphadenitis
- Psoas abscess
- Unascended kidney
- Ameboma
- Chondroma from iliac crest.

Left Iliac Fossa (LIF)
- Ca descending / sigmoid colon
- Lymph nodes
- Ovarian pathology
- Never forget in females—Uterus and Adnexia

Examination of Oral Cavity

1. Lips
2. Oral mucosa—cheek, vestibule of mouth, palate.
3. Gums
4. Retromolar trigone
5. Dental status and formula
6. Tonsils—anterior and posterior pillar
7. Posterior pharyngeal wall
8. Tongue—anterior 2/3rd and posterior 1/3rd
9. Floor of mouth
10. Stenson's duct and Wharton's duct
11. Regional lymph nodes
    - Submental
    - Submandibular
    - Preauricular
    - Upper deep cervical, etc.

Important Surgical Terms

Ablation	- The process of removal of tissue
Abscess	- Localized collection of pus walled off by damaged and inflamed tissue
Carbuncle	- Collection of boils with multiple drainage channels.
Cyst	- Abnormal sac or closed cavity is lined by epithelium or endothelium
Dysphagia	- Difficulty in swallowing
Ectomy	- Suffix denoting surgical removal of a part of all of an organ, e.g.: gastrectomy
Fistula	- Abnormal communication between two epithelial surfaces.
Furuncle	- Boils, small subcutaneous staphylococcal infection of hair follicle
Gangrene	- Putrefactive necrosis
Hematoma	- Accumulation of blood within the tissue to form a solid swelling
Induration	- Abnormal hardening of a tissue or organ
Intussusception	- Telescoping of one part of bowel with another

Itis	- Suffix denoting inflammation
Necrotic	- Dead
Obstipation	- Failure to pass flatus and stool.
Odynophagia	- Painful swallowing
Ostomy	- Any surgery of making artifical opening between the hollow organ and abdominal wall for drainage.
Otomy	- Suffix denoting surgical incision into an organ
Pexy	- Suffix denoting fixation
Pseudocyst	- Dilated cavity resembing a cyst but not lined by epithelium
Pus	- Liquid product of inflammation consist of dying leucocytes and other fluids of inflammation
Sinus	- Blind track that open to the surface
Stenosis	- Abnormal narrowing of a passage or opening
Tenesmus	- Urge to defecate with ineffectual straining (often painful)
Transect	- To divide transvesely
Ulcer	- Persistant discontinuity in any epithlial surface.

chapter 8

Important Surgical Signs and Triads

Angell's Sign :
In case of torsion testis palpation of the unaffected site reveals abnormally placed testis.

Alder's Sign :
Shifting tenderness—useful to diagnose acute appendicitis in pregnancy. Tenderness of uterine origin will shift on turning the patient to one side—in contrast to fixed point of tenderness in appendicitis.

Berry's Sign :
Absence of common carotid pulsation.

Battle's Sign :
Ecchymosis over mastoid in patients with basillar # skull.

Baid's Sign :
Palpable Ryle's tube in thin persons with pseudocyst of pancreas.

Blumberg's Sign :
Rebound tenderness in the Right iliac fossa (RIF) of the abdomen. Sign of peritonitis due to the presence of inflamed organ underneath.

Boas's Sign :
Hyperaesthesia in 9th to 11th rib area posteriorly on right side—acute cholecystitis.

Branham's Sign [Nicoladonis Sign]

	AV fistula—proximal compression causes reduction in the size of swelling, disappearance of bruit and fall in pulse rate.
Blumer's Shelf :	Metastatic deposition in rectouterine (pouch of Douglas) or in rectovesical pouch.

Bouchardt's Triad :   In gastric volvulus
1. Epigastric pain
2. Emesis
3. Inability to pass nasogastric tube

Carcinoid Triad :   In carcinoid syndrome
1. Flushing
2. Diarrhea
3. Right heart failure

Carnett's Test :   Straight leg raising test

Charcots Triad :   In Cholangitis
1. Fever with chills
2. Jaundice
3. Right hypochondriac pain

Chevostek-Weiss Sign : Tapping infront of tragus produces facial constriction (hypocalcemia).

Caput Medussae :   Radiating dilated veins from the umblicus.

Castel's Sign :   Normally splenic dullness is not elicited. If spleen is doubly enlarged, the dullness can be elicited.

Courvoisier's Law :   It is only a statement and not a law. In a jaundiced patient, if there is an enlarged non-tender gall bladder it is not due to stones (for the gall bladder will be shrunked and scarred due to chronic cholelithiasis).

It is only due to carcinoma head of pancreas.

Cullen's Sign : Bluish discoloration of periumbilical region in acute hemorrhagic pancreatitis

Cushing's Triad : In increased ICT
1. Hypertension
2. Bradycardia
3. Irregular respiration

Dalrymple's Sign : Visible upper sclera—hyperthyroid

Dance's Sign : Intussusception—ileocecal (Sign de dance).

Empty RIF with sausage shaped mass with convexity towards umbilicus—changing its position.

Dott's Sign : Differentiate pain due to basal pneumonia from appendicitis—compression of lower thorax elicite pain in lesions above diaphragm.

Fothergill's Sign : Used to differentiate infra abdominal mass on the abdominal wall.

If mass is felt while there is tension on the musculature then it is in the wall (patient sitting half-way upright).

Fox Sign : Discoloration near inguinal ligament in some cases of hemorrhagic pancreatitis.

Grey Turner's Sign :   Ecchymosis in flanks—pancreatitis.

Harvey's Sign :   Venous refilling is poor in ischemic limb and increased in AV fistula when you do Harvey's test (Two Index Fingers empty the vein on both side and release the distal finger).

Hilton's Rules of Incision (I) and Drainage (D):

1. Incision preferably in the langer's line at the maximum point of fluctuation.
2. Incision parallell to know neurovascular bundle.
3. Knife to be used only in skin beyond which sinus forcep's to be used.

Blair's modification of Hilton's method for parotid abscess: Though the skin incision is made in the parotid region vertically, the drainage is made parallel to the facial nerve course.

Homan's Sign :   Calf pain on dorsiflexion of foot in DVT (deep vein thrombosis)

Howship Ramberg's Sign :

                        Pain along the inner aspect of thigh in obturator herina due to nerve compression.

Joffroy's Sign :   Absence of wrinkling on the forehead when the patient looks upwards with the face inclined downwards (hyperthyroidism)

Kehr's Sign :   Referred pain in left shoulder due to splenic injury

Klein's Sign : Shifting tenderness in acute nonspecific mesenteric adenitis to left side on turning the patient to left lateral position in contrast to acute appendicitis.

Kenawy's Sign : Auscultation of loud venous hum beneath xiphoid process during inspiration in case of portal HT (due to splenic vein engorgement and compression).

Kelly's Sign : To identify ureter during surgery. Visible peristalsis of ureter in response to squeezing or retraction.

London's Sign : Pattern of bruising—an imprint of clothing or seat belt on the abdominal skin indicates the crushing force.
  - rupture of vessel due to crush against vertebral column.

Laplace's Law : Wall tension = Pressure × Radius
Hence colonic perforations more at cecum due to increase in radius and resultant increase in wall tension.

Larry's Point : Subxiphoid

Mcburney's Point : 1/3rd of distance from anterior superior iliac spine in the right spinoumbilical line, corresponds to base of the appendix (Manson Barr's Amoebic point is the same point on the left side).

Mittelschmerz :   - Lower quadrant ache pain due to ovulation. If on the right side, D/D for appendicitis.

Malletguy's Sign :   Patient on right lateral position with hips and knee in flexion. Deep palpation of left subcostal and epigastric region may elicit tenderness in pancreatic.

Pathology such as tumors, cyst, acute and chornic pancreatitis.

Moebius Sign :   Inability to converge eye balls (hyper-thyroidism)

Murphy's Punch :   Pressure on renal angle eliciting pain, e.g. pyelonephritis

Murphy's Sign :   Pain below the tip of the 9th costal cartilage at the peak of inspiration (in acute cholecystitis).

Murphy's Triad :   In acute appendicitis
1. Pain in right iliac fossa (RIF)
2. Fever
3. Vomiting

Obturator Sign :   Pain on internal rotation of thigh with hip and knee flexed, e.g. appendicitis and pelvic abscess.

Psoas Sign :   Pain elicited by extending hip with knee in full extension.
- Appendicitis
- Psoas inflammation

Reynold's Pentad :   Charcot's triad +
1. Mental changes
2. Shock/Sepsis in Suppurative cholangitis.

Rovsing's Sign :   LIF palpation result in pain in RIF in appendicitis.

Stellwag's Sign :   Starring look with widened palpebral fissure hyperthyroidism

Sandblom Triad :   In hemobilia
1. Melena
2. Jaundice
3. Pain

Saint's Triad :   1. Cholelithiasis
2. Hiatus hernia
3. Diverticulum

Quincke's Trial in Hemobilia
1. Right upper quadrant abdominal pain
2. Jaundice
3. UGI bleeding

Sister Mary Joseph's Sign :

Presence of metastasis in umbilical lymph node.

Tillaux Triad of Mesenteric Cyst :
1. Soft intra-abdominal swelling in the umbilical region.
2. Free mobility in a direction perpendicular to the attachment of mesentery (left side of L1, to RIF)
3. "Island of dullness in a sea of resonance"

Trousseau's Sign: BP cuff raised to 200 mm of Hg within 5 minutes contraction of hand—like obstertrician hand—

finger extended, metacarpopha-langeal joints flexion and thumb adduction.

- Parathyroid tetany— hypocalcemia

Virchow's Nodes (Troisier's Sign) :

Metastasis in the left supraclavicular node between the two heads of sternomastoid.

Virchow's Triad : Risk factor for thrombosis

1. Stasis
2. Abnormal endothelium
3. Hypercoagulation

Vas Deferens Sign : Vas can be traced behind the testis in hematocele and not in testicular tumors.

Whipple's Triad : Evidence of insulinoma:

1. Hypoglycemia
2. CNS and vasomotor symptoms like syncope, etc.
3. Relief after administration of glucose.

Important Surgical Anatomy

TRIANGLES OF IMPORTANCE

1. **Calot's Triangle :**
   - Bounded medially by common hepatic duct
   - Above by inferior border of liver
   - Below by cystic duct
   - Contents : Cystic artery, cystic lymph gland of *Lund*.

2. **Triangles of Neck :**
   a. Digastric Triangle: Inferior ramus of mandible, both digastric bellies.
   b. Submental Triangle: Anterior belly of both digastric, body of hyoid bone
   c. Carotid Triangle: Posterior belly of digastric, superior belly of omohyoid, anterior border of sternomastoid
   d. Posterior Triangle: Sternomastoid, trapezius, mid one-third of clavicle. Further divided into occipital triangle and supra- clavicular triangle by inferior belly of omohyoid.

3. **Sherren's Triangle:**
   Umbilicus, pubic symphysis, right anterosuperior iliac spine, hyper aesthesia in acute appendicitis

4. **Hasselbach's Triangle:**
   1. Inferior epigastric vessels—laterally
   2. Inguinal ligament—below
   3. Lateral border of rectus sheath medially.

INGUINAL ANATOMY

- **Deep Ring :** Defect in transversalis fascia.

  Inf. epigastric vessels medially.

  Surface marking: Half inch above mid inguinal point (mid-point of line joining anterosuprior iliac spine and pubic symphysis)

- **Superficial Ring :** Triangular defect in the external oblique aponeurosis above the pubic tubercle. Medial, lateral crura with intercrural fibres.

  Surace marking : Just above and medial to pubic tubercle.

- **Inguinal Canal:** Length : 4 cm

  Anterior wall: Skin, two layers of superficial fascia, external oblique aponeurosis, lateral one-third of fleshy fibres of internal oblique.

  Posterior wall : Fascia transversalis, medially by conjoint tendon and reflected part of inguinal ligament.

  Floor : Grooved upper surface of inguinal ligament, medially lacunar ligament.

  Roof : Arching fibres of internal oblique and transverse abdominis muscles.

Gerota's Fascia : Fascia surrounding the kidney.

PARTS OF GASTROINTESTINAL TRACT WHICH ARE RETROPERITONEAL

1. Most of duodenum
2. Ascending colon
3. Descending colon
4. Pancreas.

Interpectoral Lymph Nodes : Between pectoralis major and minor "Rotter's Node".

Morrison's Pouch : Hepatorenal recess, the most posterior cavity in the peritoneal cavity.

Foregut: Mouth to ampulla of Vater

Midgut: Ampulla of Vater to distal one-third of transverse colon.

Hindgut: Distal one-third of transverse colon to rectum.

Drainage of Left Testicular vein > Left renal vein.

Drainage of Right Testicular vien > IVC.

Blood Supply to the Breast :
- Axillary artery branches
  - Lateral thoracic (external mammary)
  - Superior thoracic artery
- Second perforating branch of internal mammary artery
- Perforating branches of posterior intercostal arteries.

Blood Supply to Appendix :
1. Appendicular artery (inferior division of Ileocaecal artery which is a branch of superior mesenteric artery)
2. Accessory appendicular artery of seshachalam.

Blood Supply to Stomach :
Along Lesser Curvature
1. Left gastric artery (from celiac trunk)
2. Right gastric artery (from hepatic artery)

Along the Greater Curvature
 i. Left gastroepiploic artery (from splenic artery)
ii. Right gastroepiploic artery (from gastroduodenal branch of hepatic artery)

   Fundus is supplied by short gastric arteries from splenic artery.

Surgical Lobes of Liver : Divided into right and left lobes by Cantle's Line

- Drawn from fossa of IVC to gall bladder bed.

  Segments I, II, III and IV - Left Lobe V, VI, VII and VIII - Right Lobe Segment I is caudate

  Lobe having independent supply of portal and hepatic veins.

Femoral Canal : Medial most compartment of the femoral sheath.

Extends from femoral ring to saphenous opening (1.25 cm.) and contains fat, lymph vessels and lymph node of cloquet.

Femoral Ring : It is an fibro-osseous ring; hence femoral hernia is more prone for strangulation.

- Anteriorly: Inguinal ligament
- Posteriorly: Public ramus and iliopectineus muscle
- Medially: Lacunar ligament
- Laterally: Femoral vein separated by a septum.

Surgical Bits

SKIN LAYERS

- **Epidermis**
  - Stratum corneum
  - Stratum lucidum
  - Stratum granulosum
  - Stratum spinosum
  - Stratum basale
- **Dermis**
- **Subcutaneous Tissue**

  Epidermis originates from the ectoderm. Other two layers develop from mesoderm.

  Few epidermal structures—pilosebaceous unit and nail matrix migrate during development and present in the dermis. Similarly some cells of mesodermal origin migrate and present in the basal layer of epidermis—melanocytes.

CARBUNCLE

- Infective gangrene of the skin and subcutaneous tissue
- Staphylococcus aureus main organism
- Nape of neck and back—main sites
- common in diabetes

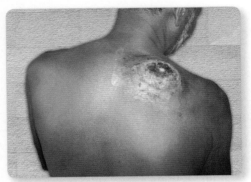

Figure 10.1: Carbuncle back

- Treatment—antibiotics—control of diabetes—drainage by cruciate incision and debridement—if needed skin graft later.

POTT'S PUFFY TUMOR

- Misnomer as it is a swelling due to subperiosteal pus and edema of scalp
- In frontal region due to osteomyelitis (OM) of frontal bone
- Due to frontal sinusitis or trauma
- Complication of extension into intracranial cavity—intracranial abscess
- Differential diagnosis (D/D)—secondaries of skull
- Treatment—antibiotics and early drainage
- Late cases need neurological decompression.

SEBACEOUS CYST

1. Retention cyst—multiple
2. Punctum Present
3. May also exist without punctum

4. Skin not pinchable
5. Treatment: Excision
6. Complications—infection, ulceration, horn
7. Ulcerated sebaceous cyst of scalp known as "cocks peculiar tumor".

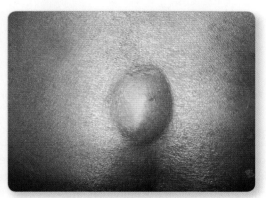

Figure 10.2: Sebaceous cyst

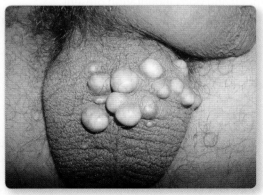

Figure 10.3: Multiple sebaceous cysts scrotum

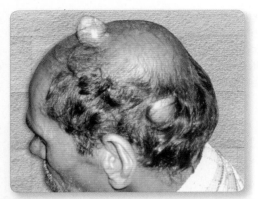

Figure 10.4: Sebaceous cysts scalp—Cock's Peculiar tumor

DERMOID CYST

Congenital, sequestrational dermoid—occurs in the line of embryonic fusion. Median nasal, external and internal auricular, preauricular, postauricular, etc.

- Skin is pinchable
- Underlying bony indentation present
- X-ray of the area must be taken to exclude intracranial extension
- Treatment—Excision

Other Dermoids

1. *Tubulo dermoid:* e.g. Thyroglossal cyst, Post anal dermoid
2. *Implantation dermoid:* In women and Tailors due to epidermal inclusion into subcutaneous tissue due to trauma.
3. *Teratomatous dermoid:* Tumor from totipotential cells.

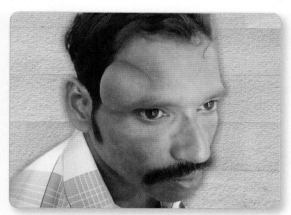

Figure 10.5: Dermoid cyst

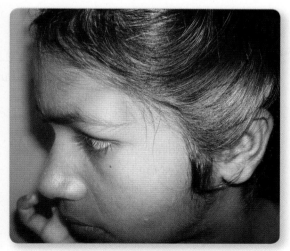

Figure 10.6: Sequestration dermoid

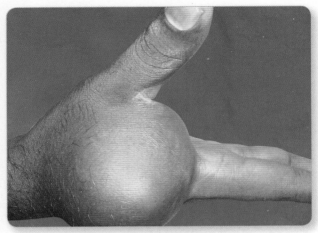

Figure 10.7: Implantation dermoid

BASAL CELL CARCINOMA (RODENT ULCER)

- Usually situated above the line joining angle of mouth and tragus.
- Slow growing—recurrent ulcer with healing and scar formation.
- Fast growing—'Field fire type'
- Edges rolled out and raised
- Locally malignant, pearl color
- No lymph node involvement
  Rx.: – Excision with skin grafting
    – If too big—Radiotherapy.

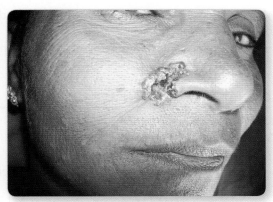

Figure 10.8: Basal cell carcinoma

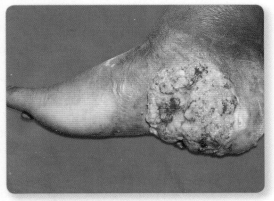

Figure 10.9: Squamous cell carcinoma

SQUAMOUS CELL CARCINOMA (EPITHELIOMA)

- Typical malignant ulcer with everted edges
- Arise from prickle cell layer
- Lymph node metastasis: Positive

- Marjolin's ulcer—malignancy from long standing burns, scar or venous ulcers.
  - As the lymphatics are destroyed early, no lymph node involvement.

MALIGNANT MELANOMA

- More common in fair people.
- 50% from pre-existing naevi
  - Junctional naevi are 90% prone
  - Present in palm, plantar aspect of foot and external genitalia.

C.F.: 1. Lentigo Maligna [Hutchinson's melanotic freckle]
  - More in face—malar region, flat, least malignant.

2. Superficial spreading melanoma (SSM)
  - Commonest; occur in trunk and exposed parts
  - Raised lesion with irregular edge.

3. Nodular Melanoma:
  - Most dangerous
  - Sites unxposed to sun—often amelanotic
  - Elevated; convex or even pedunculated.

4. Acral Lentiginous:
  - Occur in palm, sole, under nails (subungual)
  - Poor prognosis like nodular.

5. Amelanotic:
  - Worst prognosis
  - Loss of pigment especially in the centre
  - Pink in color.

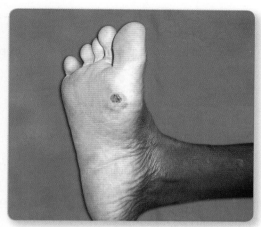

Figure 10.10: Malignant melanoma

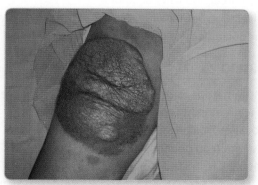

Figure 10.11: Giant hairy naevus

Classification:

- Clark's - Based on dermal layers invasion—5 types.
- Breslow - Based on thickness—4 types.

Management:

1. Confirm by biopsy
   – Excision of 1 cm margin for 1mm Breslow depth is advised.
2. Early cases
   – Wide local excision (three dimensional)
   – Defect closed by graft
   – Nodes are involved—do block dissection.
3. Advanced cases
   – Locally with distant metastases
   – Palliative chemotherapy—DTIC + Nitrosamines, BCG, Interleukin -2/Immunosuppression

Benign mole turning malignant

- Increase in Size
- Increase in intensity of color
- Ulceration or bleeding
- Irregular margins or surface elevation

GANGLION

- Myxomatous degeneration of fibrous tissue tendon sheath or joint capsule
- Localized, painless, tense, cystic swelling
- Common on dorsum of hand
- Mobility restricted along the length of tendon
- Excision under GA with bloodless field [Tourniquet]

Compound Palmar Ganglion

Chronic inflammation of common flexor sheath of tendon present below and above flexor retinaculum. Presence of "Melon Seeds" Fibrin particles. Cross fluctuation present.

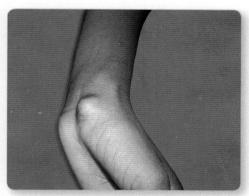

Figure 10.12: Ganglion

BURSA

- Fluid filled cavity lined with flattened endothelium similar to synovium.
- Present between tendons and bone to allow easier movement.
- Anatomical and adventitious

HEMANGIOMA (VASCULAR SWELLINGS)

- Development malformation of blood vessels—hamartomas (developmental error resulting in accumulation of different embryonic tissues)
1. Capillary
2. Cavernous—venous
3. Arterial—plexiform
4. Miscellaneous—glomus

1. Capillary—in babies
   - Salmon patch
   - Portwine stain

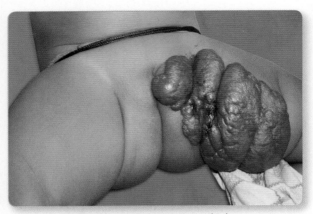

Figure 10.13: Hemangioma thigh

- Strawberry angioma
  Usually regress spontaneously

2. Cavernous
- Present since birth with no tendency for regression.
- Bluish soft swelling
- Compressible
- Non-pulsatile
- May be acquired—Post-traumatic

3. Arterial—plexiform hemangioma
- Soft red swelling
- Compressible
- Pulsatile
- Thrill and bruit present
  - *AV Fistula*
- Congenital or following trauma, surgery or in dialysis
- Compressible and pulsatile

- You may be disappointed if you fail, but you are doomed if you have not tried

- May show dilated superficial veins
  [*Arterialization of veins*]
- *Nicoladonis sign* present [refer surgical terms]
- Deep seated—diffuse hypertrophy of limbs

Complications of Hemangiomas

1. Hemorrhage
2. Ulceration
3. Infection
4. Diffuse hypertrophy of limbs

R_x: Fibrosis

   a. Hot H_2O injection
   b. Hypertonic saline
   c. Sclerosants
      - Excision
      - Selected cases of hemangioma, interventional radiological embolisation of feeding vessel causes regression.

SARCOMA

- Soft tissue turnor from tissues of mesodermal origin
- Painless, if painful due to compression of adjacent structures and stretching
- Lower limb 45%; trunk, mediastinum, retroperitoneum 30%; upper limb 15%; head and neck 10%
- Suspect sarcoma in any enlarging soft tissue mass situated deep to deep fascia
- Presence of dilated veins over the mass, warmth
- Metastasis via blood usually.

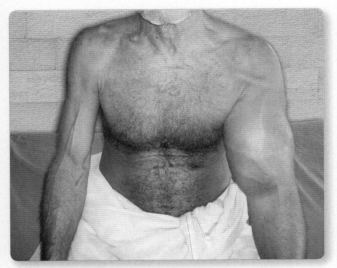

Figure 10.14: Soft tissue sarcoma—rhabdomyo

Sarcomas Spreading to Lymphnode

- Malignant Fibrous Histiocytoma
- Synovial Sarcoma
- Lympho Sarcoma
- Ewing's Sarcoma

Most Common Sarcoma in adults

- Liposarcoma, Fibrous - Histiocytoma

Most common Sarcoma in children

- Rhabdomyosarcoma, Fibrosarcoma
- TNM Staging includes histological grade also.

• Asking for help is strength not weakness

Diagnosis:

MRI / CT

FNAC

- Less than 3 cm—Excisional biopsy.
- more than 3 cm—Incisional biopsy.

R_x: Wide excision - Compartmentectomy, etc.

- Amputation last resort
- Surgery with radiation good result.
- Palliation with chemotherapy
- Adriamycin and Ifosfamide

CARCINOMA OF ORAL CAVITY

- Carcinoma of tongue and carcinoma of cheek commonly
- Ulcer or ulceroproliferative lesion

Remember the Predisposing Factors

- Smoking
- Spirit
- Sharp tooth
- Sepsis
- Spicy food
- Susceptability
- Syphilis (rare now)
- Sideropenic dysphagia (Plummer Vinson Syndrome)
- Look for Leukoplakia
  - Cracked white paint appearance
  - 'Raw Beef' appearance

Definte Premalignant Condition

- Leukoplakia
- Erythroplakia
- Chronic hyperplastic candidiasis

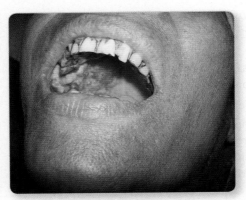

Figure 10.15: Carcinoma of oral cavity

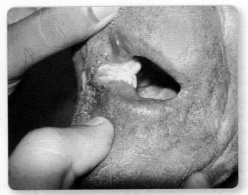

Figure 10.16: Carcinoma of cheek

Intermidiate Precursors

- Oral submucous fibrosis
- Syphilitic glossitis
- Sideropenic dysphagia

- Not just 'Go' through life, but 'Grow' through life

Some Doubtful Conditions
- Oral lichenplanus
- Discoid lupus erythematosus
- Dyskeratosis congenita
- Examine the drainage lymph node

R$_x$: Surgery
   Radiotherapy

RANULA

- Retention cyst of sublingual glands, glands of Blandie and Nuhn
- Bluish translucent swelling underneath the tongue.

Plunging Ranula

- Ranula extending into sub-mandibular region.
- Bidigitally palpable.

Treatment

- Excision or Marsupialisation.

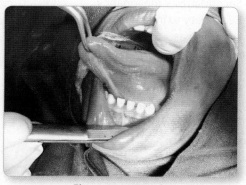

Figure 10.17: Ranula

- 'Impossible' is a word only in the dictionary of fools - Napolean

EPULIS

- Swelling over the gums arising from mucoperiosteum.
- Granulomatous—due to infection and dentures.

Rx: Scrap and treat the cause

- Fibrous—due to fibroma or fibrosarcoma of periodontal membrane

Rx: Tooth extraction + Wedge resection of bone and gum.

- Giant Cell Epulis—osteoclastoma of jaw.
- X-ray—pseudotrabeculation and bone destruction.

Rx: Radical resection of jaw.

- Carcinomatous—epithelioma of gum—invades and destroys the bone.

Rx: Wide resection/Radiotherapy.

CERVICAL LYMPHADENOPATHY

- Commonest cause of swelling in the neck
  1. TB adenitis
  2. Secondaries—malignancy
  3. Secondary to infective foci
  4. Lymphomas

Stages of TB Cervical Nodes
  1. Discrete nodes
  2. Periadenitis—matted nodes
  3. Caseation—Cold abscess
  4. TB sinus

Secondaries Neck
  1. Hard nodes—assess the mobility
  2. Search for primary—tongue, cheek etc.

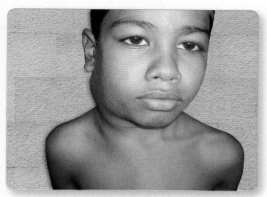

Figure 10.18: Cervical lymphadenitis

3. Occult primary are regions not accessible to routine Clinical examination

- Fossa of rosenmuller
- Vallecula
- Pyriform sinus
- Post cricoid
- Cricopharynx

FILARIAL LEG

Cold and swollen leg, warm if associated with lymphangitis.

Clinical Staging

i. Lymphoedema, less than 2 cm difference in circumference between two limbs—pitting.
ii. Difference 2–5 cm, pitting
iii. Non pitting edema, no skin changes.
iv. Non pitting edema with skin changes.

• Be a good listner, your ears will never get you in trouble

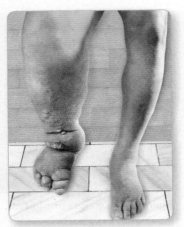

Figure 10.19: Filarial leg

R$_x$: Stage I and II:

- Elastocrepe bandaging
- Compression—chambers
- Massive Penicillin—long acting
- Nodovenous shunt Operation
- Diethyl Carbamazine—100 mg TDS for 3 days,
- Repeated every 15 days

Stage III and IV: Total excision and skin grafting *Swiss Roll*
operation

CARCINOMA OF PENIS

- Ulcer or ulceroproliferative lesion involving glans penis
- Look for extension into shaft
- Assess lymph nodes status—inguinal
- Usually squamous cell carcinoma
- Rarely BCC, malignant melanoma and adenocarcinoma
from Tyson's glands

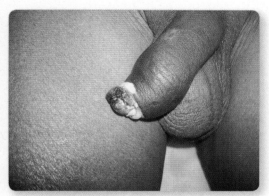

Figure 10.20: Carcinoma Penis

- Predisposing conditions
  - Chronic balonoposthitis
  - Leukoplakia
  - Erythroplasia of querat (Paget's disease)
  - Multiple papilloma
  - Giant condyloma acuminatum (Busche-Lowenstein tumor)
- Biopsy
- Total amputation of penis with perineal urethrostomy
- If adequate shaft is not involved—partial amputation
- Radiotherapy
- Block dissection of involved lymph nodes.

LYMPHOMA

HODGKIN'S	**NON-HODGKIN'S**
1. Bimodal age group	4th decade
2. Nodal 90%	Nodal 60%
Extranodal 10%	Extranodal 40%

• Learn to see, to hear, to feel and to smell—that is clinical method

3. Mediastinum Involvement	±
4. Waldeyer's ring	±
5. Epitrochlear node	±
6. GIT	±
7. Bone marrow	±
8. Centripetal	Centrifugal
9. Contiguity spread	Noncontiguity
10. Cells of origin	

- Monocytic macrophage
  Mostly B cell reticular cell

ANN ARBOR CLASSIFICATION

Stage I: Involvement of one lymph node region

I_E: One extralymphatic site or organ

II: Two lymph node groups on the same side of diaphragm.

II_E: One or more lymph node groups with one extralymphatic site on the same side of diaphragm.

III: Lymph node groups on both side of diaphragm, involvement of spleen

III_E: One extra lymphatic site on both sides of diaphragm.

IV: Diffuse or disseminated involvement of extralymphatic sites or organs.

Rye's modification of Luke and Butler Classification:

1. Lymphocyte predominant - I
2. Nodular sclerosis - II and III
3. Mixed cellularity - II and III
4. Lymphocyte depletion - IV

R_x: Radiotherapy for stage I, II and III 3500–4000 rads preferably by *Linear Accelerator*

- Chemotherapy for stage III_E and IV

- MOPP —Mustard, Vincristine, Prednisolone and Procarbazine
- ABVD—Adriamycin, Bleomycin, Vincristine and Dacarbazine.

ULCERS

- Persistent breach in the continuity of any epithelial surface.
- Describe the Ulcer in terms of size, shape, site, margins, edge, floor (visible part within Ulcer) and base (the tissue on which the Ulcer is situated) palpated.
- Discharge from the Ulcer.
- Regional lymph nodes.
- Look for zones of healing:

White Zone: Outer fibrous zone containing fibroblasts and vessels.

Blue Zone: Middle zone with multiple layers of veins with epithelal covering.

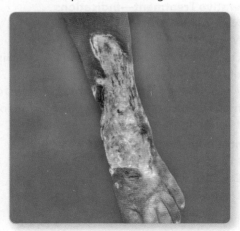

Figure 10.21: Chronic ulcer

Crimson (Red) Zone: Inner zone with a single layer of vessels with epithelial covering.

1. **Malignant Ulcers:** Basal cell carcinoma and squamous cell carcinoma and malignant melanoma.

2. **Venous Ulcers:**
   - In varicose veins and postphlebitis.
   - Usually in the lower one-third of leg—medial aspect.
   - Irregular ulcer on a bony base.
     R_x: Daily dressings with compression bandages— Bisgaurd Regimen
   - 4 Layer bandage
     - Wool
     - Crepe
     - Elastocrepe and
     - Adhesive outer wrap.
   - Antiseptic cleansing and elastic compression bandage
   - Suitable Antibiotics.

   Operative Treatment—indications
   - No response to medical management
   - Multiple
   - Large ulcer diameter more than 2.5 cm. with area of Lipodermosclerosis 5 cm.
   - Associated saphenofemoral or perforator incompetence must be treated prior to Ulcer treatment.

   Contraindications:
   1. Infection
   2. Diffuse edema of skin
   3. Deep vein obstruction

Surgical Procedures:

1. Dodd's subfascial ligation
2. Cockett's suprafascial ligation
3. Linton's procedure—excision of ulcer and grafting

3. **Arterial Ulcers**
   - Signs of ischemia present
   - Absence of pulses
   - Variable in size and shape
   - Punched out edges
   - Usually in toes, dorsum of feet and heel.

4. **Neuropathic (Trophic) Ulcers**
   - Commonly due to Diabetes Mellitus (With Vascular insufficiency and repeated infection)
   - Other Causes - Spina bifida, Leprosy, Alcoholic polyneuritis, Tabes Dorsalis etc.
   - Painless, Non tender, Deeply penetrating, punched out
   - Surrounding tissue healthy but loss of sensation may be present
   - Sole, heel of foot (Pressure Areas)

AINHUM

- Idiopathic gangrene appearing as a fissure in the interphalangeal joint of little toe followed by appearance of a fibrous band. This encircles the digit leading to necrosis.

Treatment

- Z plasty
- If fails do amputation

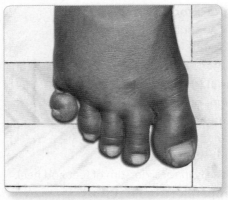

Figure 10.22: Ainhum

PYOGENIC GRANULOMA

- Small, raised, pedunculated soft red nodular lesion
- Show superficial ulceration and tends to bleed with trivial trauma
- Histologically shows features of hemangioma
- Excise with minimal margin.

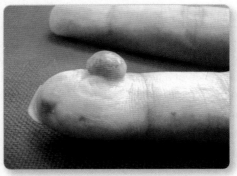

Figure 10.23: Pyogenic granuloma

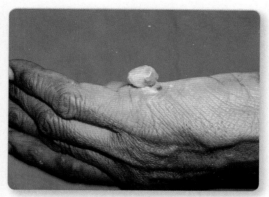

Figure 10.24: Pyogenic granuloma

SCARS

Scar is a metabolically active and dynamic tissue

- Stage 1: 0–4 weeks—soft, fine and weak scar
- Stage 2: 4–12 weeks—red, hard and strong scar
- Stage 3: 12–40 weeks—soft, white and supple scar

Peculiarities of scar formation

- Scar remodeling—process of reorientation of collagen fibres—may continue for up to one year or more
- During maturation, type III collagen converted to type I collagen
- At the time of suture removal wound strength is minimal—about 10–15%
- Rapid increase in strength after 4 weeks till 3 months
- Phenomenon of over healing leads to *hypertrophic scar* and *keloid*
- Wound contraction is essential component in scar formation—central granulation tissue theory and picture frame theory.

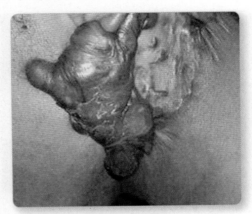

Figure 10.25: Keloid

Keloid

- Common in negroid and TB patients
- Familial tendency and more prevalent in females
- Characterised by proliferation of immature fibroblasts and immature blood vessels
- Grow beyond margins of the wound
- Ugly, pink, smooth surfaced, raised patches with claw-like processes
- Typically get worse even after a year.

Treatment

- Prevention better than care
- Careful incisions in sternum, shoulders and back—prone for Keloids
- Incisions are best made in Langer's line—lines of skin tension
- Intralesional triamcinolone—40 mg/mL—2 mL used in single sitting to be repeated after 6–8 weeks. Response 31% to 100%

- Surgical excision hazardous
- Elastic compression bandage and silicone sheet—by pressure effect
- Interstil radiotherapy
- Oral antihistamines for itching.

Comparison

Hypertrophic Scar	Keloid
- M:F equal	- F>M
- Not familial	- May be familial
- Not related to race	- More in black population
- Affects children	- 10–30 years
- Remains within wound margin	- Goes beyond wound margin into normal tissues
- No regression after 6 months	- Progressive even after 1 year
- No itching	- Usually itches
- Nontender with normal vascularity	- Tender with increased vascularity
- Common in abdomen and joints.Flexor surface usually affected	- Common in sternum, shoulders and back

PSEUDOCYST OF PANCREAS

H/O • Attacks of pain followed by appearance of swelling usually in the epigastrium in known alcoholic patient.

O/E • Globular swelling in epigastrium
- Usually not moving with respiration
- Intra-abdominal—retroperitoneal
  Baid's Sign—palpable Ryle's tube in thin abdomen

Pathology

- Collection of inflammatory exudate in the lesser sac following an attack of pancreatitis due to duct disruption
- Walled off - (no true cyst with epithelial lining).

• All surgeries are major and there is no minor surgery

Investigation
- US/CT Abdomen
- Barium meal lateral view show increased pre-vertebral shadow with stomach pushed anteriorly.

Treatment
- Wait for 4–6 weeks—usually resolves 20–50%
- Indications for surgery
  1. Non-resolving pseudo cyst.
  2. Rapidly enlarging
  3. Cyst with complications
- Infection
- Obstruction - CBD -> Jaundice
- Hemorrhage
- Rupture

Internal Drainage: Cystogastrostomy or any near by viscera—duodenum or jejunum.

External Drainage: Under US Guidance

RENAL LUMPS

1. Hydronephrosis kidney
2. Renal cell carcinoma
3. Polycystic kidney

Characters
1. Renal angle fullness
2. Reinform shape
3. Doesnot cross mid line (usually)
4. Moves with respiration
5. Bimanually palpable and ballotable
6. Upper margin could not be made out

• Never surrender your dreams to negative thoughts

7. Insinuation of fingers between lump and costal margin is possible
8. Lower pole is palpable
9. Dull on percussion with a band of colonic resonance

Hydronephrosis

- Smooth, tensely cystic, non tender renal lump
- H/O Dietl's Crisis - Intermittent appearance of lump which disappears with passing of large quantity of Urine.

Investigation: US. IVU, Isotope renography

R_X: Anderson Hynes Pyeloplasty

Renal Cell Carcinoma

- H/O painless, profuse, periodic, hematuria
- Dull, continous, fixed renal pain
- Fever, Weight loss, anemia, HT
- Hard painless renal lump with irregular surface.
- Arise from proximal convuluted tubalar epithelium.

Classical Triad

1. Hematuria
2. Renal pain
3. Renal mass

Investigation:

- IVU, RGP, US, CT Scan
- Renal vein and IVC may be involved
- IVC involvement is not a contraindication for surgery.

R_X: Radical Nephrectomy:

- Kidney
- Perinephric fat
- Gerota's Fascia

- Adrenal gland
- Regional lymph nodes.

Advanced Causes:

- Chemo-hormonal and radiotherapy
- Vinblastine, Progesterone and androgen, nitrosourea.

Polycystic Kidney

- Genetic - autosomal dominant trait
- Family history of loss of first degree relative in young age due to HT
- H/O recurrent UTI—pain, hematuria, hypertension
- O/E lobulated smooth renal lump may be bilateral and involve liver also.

Investigation:

- US/CT Scan
- Urine—clear with low specific gravity.

Treatment

- Advise to drink lot of water, low protein diet
- Antibiotics and iron supplementation
- Rovsing's operation—puncturing cyst to relieve compression of functioning renal tissue
- Nephrectomy and transplantation

MIXED PAROTID TUMOR

- *Pleomorphic Adenoma*
- Painless swelling, slow growing present for months and years.
- Site—infront, below and behind the ear lobule. Obliterating the normal hollow behind the ramus of mandible. Typically raise the ear lobe upwards
- Well-defined edge

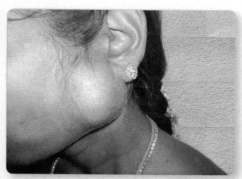

Figure 10.26: Parotid swelling

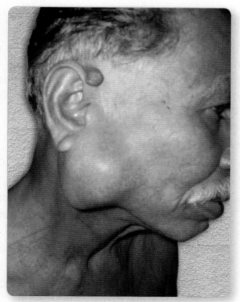

Figure 10.27: Malignant parotid tumor

- There are no regrets in life just lessons

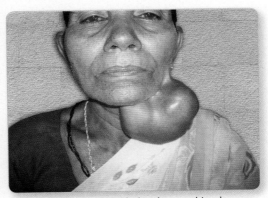

Figure 10.28: Submandibular pleomorphic adenoma

- Variable in consistency
- Skin pinchable
- Mobility and fixity to masseter to be made out by clenching the teeth
- Examine the oral cavity for Stensen's duct and involvement of deep lobe pushing the tonsillar fossa medially
- Facial nerve—normally functioning
- Rarely turn into malignancy.

D/D 1. Preauricular lymph node—its mobility distinguishes

2. Upper deep cervical—deep to sternomastoid

   – Pleomorphic adenoma is the commonest benign tumor of parotid.

   – It is called the mixed tumor because of mixed cellularity of origin—stroma formed by pseudocartilage, lymphoid and myxomatous tissue.

Diagnosis: By US/CT Scan, FNAC

R$_x$: Superficial conservative Parotidectomy (facial nerve conserved)

Complications of Surgery:

1. Flap necrosis
2. Facial nerve injury
3. Fistula formation
4. Frey syndrome.

LIPOMA - (UNIVERSAL TUMOR)

- Benign neoplasm from fat cells
- Soft, with slippery edges (slip sign)
- Lobulated
- Site: Subcutaneous, sub-fascial, inter-muscular, subserous, submucous, infra-articular, sub-synovial, parosteal, Extradural, Intra-glandular.
- Dercum's disease: Painful multiple lipomatosis.

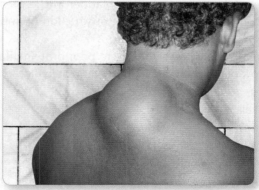

Figure 10.29: Lipoma back

Complications:
1. Enlarge in size
   - Cosmetic disfigurement and pressure effects.
2. Degenerative changes
   - Myxomatous degeneration
   - Mummification
   - Saponification
   - Calcification
3. Sarcomatous changes
4. Rare life threatening complication
   - Submucous lipoma of intestine causing Intussusception

R_x: Excision—Biopsy

VESICAL CALCULUS

Stones in the urinary bladder
- Primary—originates in the kidney and passes to bladder where it enlarges—urine is sterile
- Secondary—forms within bladder in the presence of infection, bladder outlet obstruction or impaired bladder emptying
- Were widely prevalent due to poor protein intake—now diminished due to improvement in diet.

Types
- Oxalate
- Uric acid
- Cystine
- Triple phosphate

Clinical features
- Male:female—8:1

- Experience teaches slowly at the cost of mistake

- Frequency, strangury, terminal hematuria or acute retension of urine
- Strangury seen in patients with oxalate calculus
- Severe pain referred to tip of penis or *labia majora* at the end of micturition
- Symptoms of UTI.

Investigations

- Urine—reveals hematuria, pyuria and crystals of stone present (envelope-oxalate and hexagonal –cystine)
- X-ray KUB
- Cystoscopy—definite procedure both for diagnosis and treatment.

Treatment

- Underlying cause to be treated
- BPH –prostatectomy should be done
- Endoscopy treatment is nowadays preferred Litholapaxy: stone crushed endoscopically; fragments evacuated by Ellick evacuator
- Percutaneous suprapubic litholapaxy—similar to percutaneous nephrolithotomy
- Open surgery
- ESWL.

NEUROFIBROMA

- Peripheral nerve is covered by Endoneurium, Perineurium and Epineurium
- Neurofibroma arises from these nerve sheath mostly from endoneurium
- Types: Localized (or) solitary, Generalised or von Recklinghausen's disease

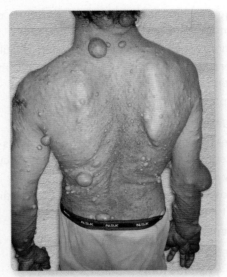

Figure 10.30: von Recklinghausen's disease

- Encapsulated round swelling of the nerve, smooth, firm, moves side ways, not along the nerve axis
- Generalised type is transmitted as autosomal dominant
- Associated with acoustic neuroma, pheochromocytoma.

Complications:

- Cystic degeneration
- Pressure effect
- Sarcomatous change

R$_x$: Observation, if complicates—excision

SCHWANNOMA (NEURILEMMOMA)

- Arises from schwann cells
- Ectodermal in origin

• Surgery is easy to watch, difficult to do

- Benign, well-encapsulated tumor
- Site—acoustic nerve, peripheral nerve, retroperitoneum, posterior mediastinum.
- Single firm, round mass
- No risk of malignant transformation.

R$_x$: Excision of tumor

THYROGLOSSAL CYST

It is an congenital anomoly, occurs due to unobliteration of thyroglossal duct.

- Become evident in the late teens
- Site: – Foramen cecum (rare)
  - Suprahyoid
  - Sub-hyoid (common)
  - At thyroid cartilage
  - At cricoid cartilage

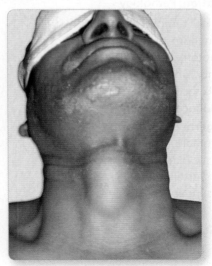

Figure 10.31: Thyroglossal cyst

- Moves with deglutition and on protruding the tongue out

R$_X$: Sistrunk operation—removal of tract with body of hyoid bone

Complication: Infection, Abscess formation, Fistula, Papillary Carcinoma

TESTICULAR TUMORS

1% of all male malignancies.

Predisposing Causes: Genetic—High-risk in men with family H/O

- Cryptorchism
- Testicular Atrophy
- HIV Infection
- H/O Previous testicular tumor

Classification: Pathology

- Germ cell tumor—about 90%
  - Seminoma
  - Teratoma
  - Embryonal cell
  - Yolk sac
  - Choriocarcinoma
- **Non-germ cell tumor**
  - Stromal
    - Leydig cell
    - Sertoli cell
  - Secondary
    - Metastatic

Clinical Staging

Stage I - Tumor testis with no metastasis

Stage II -   Metastasis continued to abdominal nodes.

Stage III - Involving supra - and inform diaphragmatic lymph nodes

Stage IV -   Extralymphatic metastasis.

Clinical Features

- Painless mass testis usually (may become painful due to hge, necrosi or truama)
- Secondary hydrocoele
- Loss of Testicular Sensation
- Rarely teratoma present with gynecomastia.

Investigations

- Estimation of serum alphafeto protein (AFP) and the beta subunit of human chorionic gonadotrophins (hCG) before any surgery
- Testicular US
- Xray chest, IVP
- CT Scan of lungs, liver and retroperitoneum

R_x: High Orchidectomy via inguinal incision with soft clamp at the deep ring level in the cord.

Subsequent management depends on histological type and staging of the tumor.

Seminoma:

- Arises from seminiferous tubules
- Low grade malignancy
- Age: 35 to 45 years
- Small and smooth on cut section.
- Lymphatic spread more
- Radiosensitive

- Finding fault is easier. Finding remedy is the one which is difficult

Teratoma:

- Arise from primitive germ cells
- May have cartilage, bone, muscle, fat, etc.
- Variable in size and in cut-section
- Age: 25 to 35 years
- Blood stream spread
- Not radiosensitive

Complications of Blood Transfusion/Massive Transfusion

- Massive transfusion is defined as transfusion of blood equivalent to the circulating blood volume within 24 hrs period
- In practice 10–12 units in adult(one unit 320 to 400 mL of blood)

Complications of Ordinary Transfusion

- Mismatch reactions
  - Hemolysis
    Hemoglobinuria
    Acute renal failure jaundice DIC
- Allergic reactions
- Transmission of various infections
- Air embolism
- Thrombophlebitis

Complications of Massive Transfusion

- Due of bulk of transfusion
  - CCF
    Pulmonary edema
    DIC (due to dilutional thrombocytopenia)
- Due to low temperature of rapidly transfused blood—arrhythmia, cardiac arrest

- RBC dysfunction(poor O_2 delivery) bleeding tendency due to thrombocytopenia and lack of factors V and VIII
  - Hyperkalemia
  - Hypocalcemia
    - increased acid load and fall in blood pH due to lactic acid content

DENTIGEROUS CYST

- Odontogenic cyst
- Occur around III molar region
- Cystic swelling covering the crown
- X-ray—unerupted tooth within cyst outer table expansion (inner table is strong)
- Treatment—removal of offending tooth and entire epithelial lining

AMELOBLASTOMA/ ADAMANTINOMA/EVES TUMOR

- Odontome
- Epithelial tumor arising from enamel forming cells
  - Ameloblasts
- Locally invasive solid tumor; may undergo multicentric cystic degeneration
- CF: painless lower jaw swelling

III decade "egg shell crackling" of outer table of mandible

- X-ray—large loculae with honey combing
- Treatment—resection of mandible with healthy margin

MAGNETIC RESONANCE IMAGING (MRI)

- Harmless procedure without ionizing radiation. Images of hydrogen nuclei throughout the body (H+most magnetic nucleus of elements; makes up two-third of atoms in all living tissues)

- MRI scanner consists of a magnet with a field strength of 20,000 times that of earth magnetic field .This makes the hydrogen ions to realign its polarity,this change in alignment causes the nucei to emit the absorbed energy as radio waves—detected by a short wave antenna and receiver and converted to images
- Details of tissue consistency made by measuring 'relaxation time'—the rate at which the signals from H+fades after stimulation.

Advantages
1. Can scan in any plane
2. Bone can be suppressed and stuctures embedded in bone such as inner ear,spinal canal,pituitary fossa can be visualized.

Disadvantages
1. Expensive
2. Time consuming
3. Not suitable for patients with metallic implants or pace makers.

COMPUTERIZED TOMOGRAPHY (CT)

- A slit of X-ray beam is directed at points on the circumference of a narrow transverse section of the body. These rays fall sequentially on multiple scintillation crystal detectors with photomultipiers—fed into a computer which builds the picture of the section examined—picture can be stored or printed
- Discrimination can be improved by IV contrast—iodine containing dyes

---

• Success is never final and failure is never fatal

- *Helical or spiral CT*—recent innovation—involves continuous rotation of X-ray tube tracing a spiral path around the patient. A single breath hold up to 30 seconds help to cover 30 cm of tissue in a single acquisition. Hence useful in children and debilitated patients(CT needs suspended respiration)other advantages are:
  1. Reduced scan time
  2. Imaging peak levels of contrast—arterial and venous phase
  3. Multiplaner and three-dimentional analysis—CT angiography,coplex joints,facial bones—virtual endoscopy of bronchial tree,colon etc.

Indications:
1. Trauma—head injury, chest injury, abdominal injury (no contrast)
2. Neoplasms—location, size, vascularity, extent and operability
3. Inflammatory conditions—psoas abscess, pseudocyst of pancreas
   - Dose of radiation similar to routine radiology

ULTRASOUND

- A non-invasive,quick and reliable investigation— inexpensive
- Ultrasound contain waves with frequency more than 20,000 cycles per second—not audible to human ear
- Principle: Tissues vary in their capacity to absorb sound. When an ultrasound wave(2–10 MHz)strikes the interface between two media of different acoustic impedance, some energy is reflected as ultrasound echo,this is recorded by a detector and displayed.

- A-Mode: Only one dimensional static display—used in eye scan
- B-Mode: Two dimensional real time images of grains, most widely used
- M-Mode:Images recorded as dots,used in moving parts—Echocardiography
- Combined with Doppler-Duplex scanning.

Uses:

1. All abdominal and pelvic conditions
2. Thyroid—to distinguish solid and cystic lesions
3. Testicular tumors,epididymo-orchitis
4. Breast to distinguish solid and cystic tumors
5. Soft tissue and musculoskeletal US
6. Very useful in gall bladder – stones well seen with acoustic shadow
   - Drawbacks: Interpretor dependent, bowel shadow may prevent proper visualisaton, inadequate image in obese
   - Advanced US—Endoultrasonography (EUS) Transvaginal, Transrectal
   - Therapeutic use—to guide aspiration in amebic liver abscess,pericardial tapping.On table to assess operability of tumor

RADIONUCLIDE IMAGING

- Represents function of an organism than morphology. Radionuclide particles emit alpha, beta and gamma rays.The gamma rays are used for diagnostic purposes mapped by gamma camera
- Technetium 99 m is the commonly used radionuclide (99 is the mass number and m-metastable) adminstered IV-short half life,emits pure gamma rays

- Other radionuclide used—Thallium201 chloride-cardiac image Gallium 67 nitrate-tumor and inflammation I$_{123}$
- Safer,easier and no side effects.

Uses:

1. Detect pulmonary emboli—Tc 99 labelled serum albumin
2. Labelled phosphate to study bone
3. Labelled sulphur—function of liver, spleen, marrow
4. Labelled HIDA—hepatocytes and biliary tracts
5. Labelled DMSA—renal functions
6. Labelled DTPA—study GFR
   Disadvantage: availability, cost, fast half life

DOPPLER STUDY-DUPLEX SCANNING

- Doppler effect is a change in the perceived frequency of sound emitted by a moving source. So it measures blood flow, combined spectral Doppler wave and Ultrasound imaging is Duplex scanning.
- Doppler provides both audio and video signals, waves may be continuous or pulsed
- Color Doppler imaging displays flowing blood towards transducer as red and as blue when away from transducer
- Reliable and noninvasive—replacing veno and angiograms
- Uses: Study CVS, vascularity of tumors, find DVT, varicose veins, perforator incompetance, to study blood flow and velocity in arterial disease—TAO, A-V fistula,cervical rib, aneurysm.

• We do not see things as they are, we see them as we are

POSITRON-EMISSION TOMOGRAPHY (PET)

- Noninvasive diagnostic method to assess the biochemical and physiological status of a tissue.used in complimentary with CT and MRI
- Two protons are used,positive electrons (positrons). Flurodeoxy glucose is commonly used
- Principle of 'Electronic collimation' is used to produce images from emitted radiation from positrons.

Uses:

1. To assess myocardial perfusion
2. Temporal lobe epilepsy to localize
3. Cancer imaging in lungs, colorectal cancer, head and neck and breast cancer,thyroid cancer ,musculoskelatol tumors

Advantage: Very specific

Disadvantage: Very expensive and limited availability.

LYMPHANGIOGRAPHY

- Investigation to evaluate the gross anatomy of peripheral lymphatics
- Steps: 5 mL of equal mixture of methylene blue and1% xylocaine injected into webspace

↓

Bluish discoloration of dermal lymphatics

↓

Cannulation by 27–30 G needle injection of contrast—Ethiodol 10 mL for leg - 5 mL for arm

---

- If someone is greedy, bribe him; if someone is foolish advice him; if someone is wise listen to him
- Difficulties are mirror on the wall, that show a person what they are in reality

Multiple x-rays in 24 hours
- Complications: Lymphangitis, contrast allergy, wound infection, arthralgia, rarely pulmonary embolisation of contrast.

ENDOSCOPY

- Viewing the interior of viscera or body cavities by instruments introduced by natural or created orifices
- Contrast to early rigid scopes now fibroptic flexible endoscopes are used. Light is transmitted by thousands of fine glass fibres coated with an opaque medium
- There is facility for irrigation, suction, tissue biopsy and photography
- Endoscopes are used for diagnosis as well as therapeutic intervention—introduction of stents
- ERCP done using side viewing endoscope.

ENDOSCOPIC RETROGRADE CHOLANGIOPANCREATOGRAPHY

- Through side viewing endoscope ampulla of Vater— sphinctor of oddi cannulated. Bile ducts visualised— bile taken for cytological and microscopic examination. Brushings can be taken from structures if needed. Water soluble dye injected and X-rays taken
- Indications: malignancy, chronic pancreatitis, stones, stricture of biliary tree, choledochal cyst, sampling bile and pancreatic juice, brush biopsy.

Therapeutic:

1. Extraction of stone from biliary tree
2. Nasobiliary drainage
3. Stenting for tumor in CBD or pancreas

4. Dilatation of biliary stricture
5. Endoscopic papillotomy

Complications: Pancreatitis, duodenal injury, cholangitis, bleeding

- MRCP—now the standard investigation for biliary tree. No need for contrast or endoscopy. MRI with appropriate computing gives a clear outline of biliary tree,but only diagnostic. T_1 images for pancreas and T_2 images for biliary tree.

MAGNETIC RESONANCE CHOLANGIO PANCREATOGRAPHY (MRCP)

- MRI imaging of biliary tract without contrast agent
- But by using contrast (IV Gadolinum—hepatocyte specific agent entirely excreted in bile), additional information of liver and pancreas can be made out
- Principle based on T_2 relaxation time pulse sequence.

Clinical Applications

1. Choledocholithiasis—95–100% sensitive
   - Detect stones as small as 2 mm
   - Detect intrahepatic stones
   - Replace ERCP in gall stones associated with acute pancreatitis
   - Can differenciate CHD obstruction by Mirrizi syndrome from GB cancer/enlarged lymph nodes.
2. Failed/incomplete ERCP
   - Useful in cases of difficulty in positioning for ERCP such as cervical spine fractures, head and neck tumors
   - Useful in altered anatomy—Billroth II, periampullary diverticula, etc.

3. Congenital anomalies
   - Choledochal cysts, annular pancreas, aberrant bile duct,abnormal pancreatico biliary junction
4. Postoperative anatomy study
   - Assess patency of hepaticojejunostomy following surgery for high bile duct stricture/hilar cholanjiocarcinoma
5. Primary sclerosing cholanjitis
6. Bile duct injuries
7. Bile duct tumors
8. Pancreatic diseases to visualize main pancreatic duct.

Advantages

Entirely noninvasive, absolutely no irradiation, image in any plane without monitoring patient, no biological hazard, no starvation required, time less taken—10 minutes.

Disadvantages

As in any MRI such as use of metallic clips, pace maker, claustrophobia.

MRCP versus ERCP

Lower failure rate, noninvasive, useful in altered/pathological anatomy.

CAPSULE ENDOSCOPY

Recent tool of investigation for GI Tract
Video imaging of the natural propulsion of a capsule through the digestive system.

Main Components

1. An indigestible capsule
2. Portable data recorder
3. Work station equipped with image processing software.

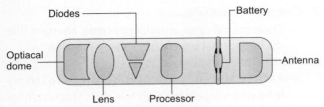

Figure 10.32: Endoscopy capsule

Capsule consists of an optical dome, lens, two emitting diodes, a processor, a battery and an antenna all within a large vitamin pill sized capsule

Uses

1. Good visualization from mouth to colon
2. Localized cryptic and occult GI bleed
3. Small bowel Crohn's disease

Contraindications

1. Small bowel stricture
2. Severe gastroparesis
3. Pseudo obstruction

Advantage:

1. No sedation
2. Painless

Disadvantages:

1. No biopsy
2. Not controllable
3. No accurate location
4. Incomplete studies due to battery life
5. Large capsule to swallow

ENDOLUMINAL ULTRASOUND

- A transducer is attached to the distal tip of the endoscope
- Five layers of gastric wall identified and depth of invasion of tumor correctly assessed 90% accuracy
- Enlarged L.N identified
- Liver metastasis not visualised by axial imaging can be made out.

Uses:

1. Lung cancer: Subcarinal, aortopulmonary and perioccipital lesions made out.
2. Oesophagus: Tumors, Barrets esophagus, dysplasia and varices made out.
3. Stomach: Evolution and staging of carcinoma stomach
   Gastric lymphoma—hypoechoic infiltration of deep mucosa and submucosa made out
4. Biliary tract: Staging of cholangiocarcinoma and detection of stone in CBD
5. Pancreas: Carcinoma head of the pancreas—nodal involvement made out.

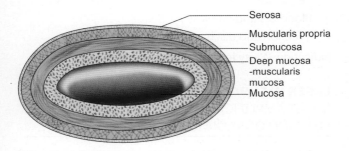

Figure 10.33: Five layers of gastric wall

STAPLERS IN SURGERY

- Used for opposition of tissues
  - skin, bowel, lungs etc
- Cutaneous staplers, linear staplers, circular staplers (End to End Anastomosing), GIA staplers for side to side anastomosis, stapler for lung apposition
- Laparoscopy surgery
  - Endostaplers and Endovascular staplers
- Hemorrhoidectomy stapler
- Technically fast and easy but cost factor and availability to be considered.

CRYOSURGERY

- Destruction of tissue by controlled cooling. system consist of a cryoprobe and defrosting device.
- Gases used—nitrous oxide, CO_2, liquid nitrogen, Freon, N_2O is cheap, easily available
- It produces intracellular crystallization, dehydration and denaturation of proteins, block microcirculation—cell death
- Bloodless and painless
- Infection and discharge are the disadvantages.

Indication: Warty lesions, piles, chronic cervicitis

LASER IN SURGERY
(LIGHT AMPLIFICATION BY STIMULATED EMISSION OF RADIATION)

- Principle: Molecules are placed in compact area and power is passed through to activate. Molecules get activated at different periods and varied directions and

each other to release energy—this is used via optical system to the desired area

- Named depending on molecule used—Argon laser, Neo-dynium Ytrium Aluminum Garnet laser(Nd-YAG laser) CO_2 laser, Neon, etc.
- Bloodless and fast
- Cost and availability are setbacks.

Uses: ENT—vocal and laryngeal leisions

Eye—retinal detachment, glaucoma

Gen surgery—bleeding duodenal ulcer, carcinoma of esophagus paliation, prostate, bladder, cervical carcinoma.

SUBDURAL HEMATOMA

- More common than EDH
- Due to laceration of brain substance and vessels—particularly cerebral veins
- Accumulation of blood in subdural space
- CT—hematoma with *Concavity* of inner surface with respect to brain
- Reason—craniotomy to remove clot and arrest of source of bleed

Chronic Subdural Hematoma

- Occurs in elderly and alcoholics because of the atrophy of brain facilitates its displacement during even trivial trauma
- Signs of cerebral compression may be delayed for weeks or months as the hematoma gradually increases due to absorption of tissue fluids by osmosis.

EXTRADURAL HEMORRHAGE: LUCID INTERVAL

- Due to disruption of middle meningeal vessels by temporal bone
- Primary brain damage often minor
- Classical h/o—transient loss of consciousness—lucid interval of apparent normalcy—then progressive deterioration of consciousness and development of coning—death
- CT—lens shaped hematoma—*convex* on its inner side
- Reason—evacuation of clot by burrhole close to fracture site with absolute hemostasis

ROBOTIC SURGERY

A remote controlled computerised tele-manipulatory system in which the three-dimensional camera system and the surgical instrumentation and manipulations are done by robotic arms which is under the control of a surgeon handling the remote switches at a distance.

Long distance use based on images via computerised electronic signals in which manual instrumentation of a surgeon is converted to electronic signal is called as *Telesurgery*.

Preparation for Robotic Surgery

- Overall fitness: Cardiac arrhythmia, emphysema
- Previous Surgery: Scars, adhesions noted
- Body habitus: Obesity, skeletal deformity
- Normal coagulation
- Thromboprophylaxis
- Informed consent.

Merits

- Endowrist with seven degree of movement
- Tremor filtration
- Effective even in small cavity
- Motion scaling in mobile organs
- Graded tip holding facilities
- Even a physically handicapped can perform surgery

Demerits

- Availability
- Time consuming
- Loss of proprioception
- Very high eye, hand and foot co-ordination needed

Robotic Systems Available

AESOP[Computer Motion, California]

Endo – Assist , UK

Da Vinci console [California]

Zeus[California]

SOCRATES [California]

FLAIL CHEST/STOVE IN CHEST INJURY

- Fracture of three to four adjacent ribs at least in two sites—floating segment of ribs which move in paradoxical manner during respiration
- Anterior flail involving sternum is known as 'stove in chest'
- There is parenchymal injury to lung
- CF: Respiratory distress—hypoxia

- Enthusiasm is the greatest asset in the world. It beats money, power and influence

- R_x aims to stabilize chest wall and reduce dead ventilatory space-good analgesics
    - Diuretics to prevent pulmonary edema
    - Minimal injury—chest physiotherapy
    - Moderate—endotracheal intubation / tracheostomy
    - Severe—tracheostomy and peep

TENSION PNEUMOTHORAX

- Occurs due to breach of visceral pleura by a fractured rib. Blunt injury chest may result in lung laceration due to fractured rib

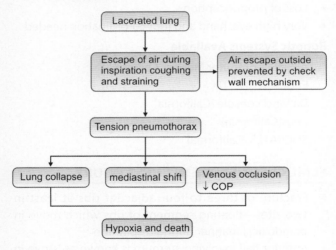

- There is generation of positive pressure in the airways due to coughing, straining, groning resulting in tension pneumothorax. Pleural space may fill with blood due to injury
- X-ray chest erect confirms—air entry in affected side; trachea pushed to opposite side

- Clinically—percussion note with diminished breath sounds
- R_x—if tension pneumo suspected, immediate treatment even before X-ray is taken—introduction of widebore needle into the affected hemithorax saves life. later chest drainage by underwater seal.

IMMUNOSUPPRESSION

- Blockage of lymphocyte proliferation in response to antigenic stimulation

Causes:

1. General disease or debilitation, e.g. diabetes mellitus, malignancy, renal and liver failure
2. Disease of immune system—AIDS, lymphoma, leukemia
   - Deliberate immunosuppression done in transplantation. Agents used are steroids, azothioprine, cyclosporin, methotrexate
   - Deliberate immunosuppression for diseases involving immune mechanisms—steroids in Crohn's disease, rhematoid arthritis, SLE
   - Splenectomy for idiopathic thrombocytopenic purpura
   - Thymectomy in myastheniagravis

Complications of Immunosuppression

- Metabolic effects—loss of appetite and lethargy
- Infections—UTI, respiratory, septicemia, viral infections
- Hematological—pancytopenia, agranulocytosis
- Dermatological—dry skin, striae, hypertrichosis
- GIT—bleed, diarrhea
- Development of tumors; skin carcinoma, lymphoma

MONOCLONAL ANTIBODIES

- By a technical process: Hybridisation myeloma cells are fused with human cells—lymphocytes.The resultant cell has capacity to multiply to produce required cell in abundance—*Hybridoma*. The monoclonal antibodies thus produced are used for
  1. Immunodiagnosis
  2. Antibody for detection of tumor antigen
  3. Cancer therapy
  4. For serotherapy

TETANUS

- Caused by *Clostridium tetani*—Anaerobic Gram positive, motile noncapsulated organism with peritrichous flagella and terminal spores (drum stick appearance)
- Spores are infective agents, found in soil, dust and manure. Enter via any wound, pricks, injuries. Established infection does little to local wound but the exotoxin produced –tetanospasmin and tetanolysin cause the damage.
- Incubation period—few days to 3 months (2 weeks usually)
- Onset time—time between first symptom to onset of muscle spasm. Shorter the time, worse the prognosis
- *Tetanospasmin* causes increased muscle tone with exaggerated response to trivial stimuli and intermittent spasms-tonic clonic convulsions.

Clinical Features

- Insiduous-tingling ache or stiffness in wound area, Lock Jaw, Risus Sardonicus, neck rigidity, dysphagia, laryngealspasm of chest wall muscle and diaphragm—respiratory difficulty.

- Opisthotonus—patient remains conscious.

Treatment

- Admit in isolated dark, quiet room
- Destruction of organism and neutralising toxin
- Human Antitetanus globulinATG 10,000 units IVdiluted in saline
- Wound debridement and excision
- Penicillin and metronidazole.

Life Support

- Sedation in quiet dark atmosphere
- Ryle's tube feeding
- Muscle relaxants
- Intubation and ventilatory support if needed.

GAS GANGRENE

- Infective gangrene caused by Clostridial organisms—*Clostridium perfringens* (*Clostridium welchii*) mainly but others *Clostridium oedematiens, septicum, histolyticus* also be associated
- *Clostridium welchii*—Gram negative, central spore bearing, nonmotile, capsulated organism—strict anerobe infection of favored by failure to debride properly
- Endotoxins – Lecithinase, collaginase, proteinase, hyloronidase
- Toxins devitalize cells, destroy microcirculation and spread via tissue planes.There is extensive necrosis of muscle with production of gas H_2S staining muscle brown black' muscle origin to insertion involved

- Liver-necrosis 'foamy liver'
- Incubation period—1 to 2 days.

Clinical feature

- Local:—crepitus, brown seropurulunt discharge and painful myositis
- Systemic:—tachycardia, pallor, cloudy consciousness
- Suspect whenever there is general deterioration of any patient with wounds
- Adequate excision and debridement can prevent myonecrosis. Avoid primary closure of dirty wounds.

Treatment

- Wide opening of wound
- Excision of devitalised tissue
- High dose of antibiotics—benzyl penicillin and metronidazole
- Hyperbaric oxygen helps to limit radical surgery
- Amputation—life saving in severe cases.

FOURNIER'S GANGRENE

- Idiopathic scrotal gangrene
- Necrotising fasciitis around male genitals—may extend to involve abdominal wall also
- Vascular disaster of infective origin
- Follows minor injuries in perineal area
- Mixed bacterial cultures grown—hemolytic streptococci with other organisms like *E. coli*, *Staphylococcus*, *Cl. welchii*.

Treatment

- Determine Hb, blood sugar, urea and electrolyte. Hemodynamic stabilization

- Intravenous antibiotics based on swab study—meanwhile combination of high-dose benzyl penicillin, metronidazole and gentamicin
- Immediate radical surgical excision of the involved area.

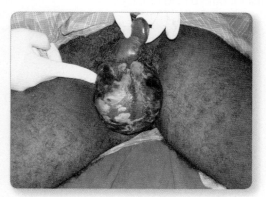

Figure 10.34: Fournier's gangrene 1

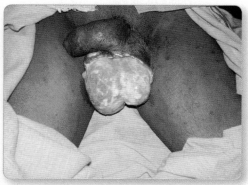

Figure 10.35: Fournier's gangrene

MYCETOMA-MADURA FOOT

- Chromic inflammatory lesion with multiple sinuses discharging granules
- Causative organisms—*Nocardia madurae, Actinomyces israeli*
- First identified in Madurai by Gill

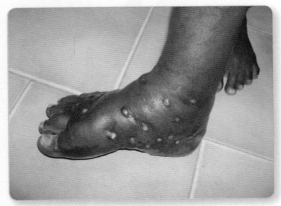

Figure 10.36: Madura mycosis

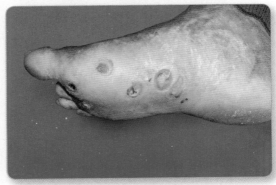

Figure 10.37: Madura mycosis

- Direct inoculation by thorn prick; 60% feet involved
- Affinity to fat and bone—muscle resistant
- Do not spread to lymph nodes unless secondary bacterial infection
- Painless diffuse swelling foot with multiple sinuses
- X-ray—moth eaten appearance of bones
- Granules viewed under microscope show sun-ray appearance.

Treatment

- Dapsone 100 mg bid+Injection SM 1 gm daily for 9 months
- Sulphamethoxone + trimethoprim + SM long-term penicillin and antifungal amphotericin.

Surgical management

- Wide excision of affected tissue under GA with
- Tourniquet for bloodless field
- Amputation only as last resort.

HYDATID DISEASE

- Caused by Tape worms—*Echinococcus granulosis* and *E. multilocularis*
- Man is accidental intermediate host. 70% occur in liver—right lobe 75%, left lobe 25%
- CF: symptomless,or present with hepatomegaly and pain; rupture may cause anaphylactic reaction. Rarely jaundice due to biliary obstruction
- Investigations: Compliment fixation test, Indirect hem-agglutination test, ELISA, US and CT X-ray may show calcification.

Medical Treatment

Indications: Extensive widespread disease

Recurrent cyst

Elderly, surgical risks, cyst ruptures and patient present with acute abdomen, albendazole therapy –good results

- Albendazole—10 mg/kg body day for one month or 40 mg Bid for 28 days—2 weeks drug free interval—3 cycles
- Praziquantel—60 mg/kg along with albendazole for 2 weeks
- Mebendazole—600 g daily for 4 weeks

Surgical Treatment

Laparotomy—protection of viscera by scolicidal agents pack—prevent spillage—use of Aarons cone, Aspiration and instillation of scolicidal agents (never in cases communicating with biliary tree)—cyst shelled out and laminated membrane removed.

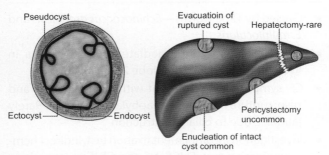

Figure 10.38: Hydatid cyst—liver

METABOLIC ALKALOSIS

- Characterised by a decrease in plasma hydrogen ion concentration and an increase in bicarbonate concentraion. A compensatory respiratory acidosis may occur with increase in partial CO_2.
- Commonly associated with hypokalemia and hypochloremia.
- Common causes in surgery: Low sodium chloride and water, vomiting, nasogastric aspiration of gastric contents, diuretics
  Hypokalemia—colorectal villous adenoma, colorectal wasting diarrhea,
  Milk alkali syndrome
- Treatment: adequate 0.9% NaCl with sufficient potassium to correct hypokalemia
- In gastric outlet obstruction initially vomiting causes dehydration; loss of potassium by kidneys result in hypokalemic metabolic alkalosis. As alkalosis worsens K stores get depleted and kidney excretes hydrogen ions—result in paradoxical aciduria.

SEPTIC SHOCK–ENDOTOXIC SHOCK

- Occur due to Gram negative bacterial infection often in strangulated intestines, peritonitis, biliary and urinary sepsis but can also occur due to Gram positive and fungus
- Endotoxin from bacterial cell wall has central importance and may be derived from organisms at site of infection or gut organisms following hypoxia/ischemic changes to mucosal barrier.

Stages:

a. Hyperdynamic (warm) shock—early reversible stage as patient is having inflammatory response based on culture, higher antibiotics.

b. Hypodynamic hypovololemic (cold) shock. Here pyogenic response is lost; patient in decompensated shock. Irreversible stage with MODS(multi organ dysfunction syndrome).

NOSOCOMIAL INFECTIONS

- Infection that becomes manifest while the patient is in hospital, typically more than 48 hrs after admission
- Infection may be endogenous—from patient own flora; or exogenous—from hospital environment; between patients, between patient and treating staff
- Prolonged stay patients acquire hospital organisms in skin, nose, mouth and gut
- Staphylococcus aureus, methicillin resistant MRSA is notorious strain of hospital origin
- Klebsiella—hospital acquired UTI
- Most of the organisms will be drug resistant, virulent, cause severe sepsis. Prevention is better by aseptic measures in wards and OT and isolating patients with severe infection
- Antibiotics—isolation—culture of blood, urine and pus to identify the causative organism
- Ventilatory support.

GASTROESOPHAGEAL REFLUX (GERD)

- Commonest cause of dyspepsia
- Caused by retrograde flow of gastric acid through an incompetent cardiac sphincter into the lower esophagus.

- CF:Reflux of acid causes inflammation and ulceration of esophageal mucosa and manifest as heart burn—retrosternal burning pain, Acid brash—regurgitation of acid content into mouth, Water brash—reflux salivation Dysphagia from benign strictures.

Management

- Investigations: Barium swallow and meal
                     OGD scopy
                     pH monitoring and esophageal manometry

- **Treatment:**
  General—raising head of bed avoid coffee, smoking, fatty food and alcohol.

  Medical—H$_2$ blockers, proton pump inhibitors, alginates to coat esophagus and prokinetic agents to improve lower esophageal muscle tone and promote gastric emptying.

  Antireflux surgery indicated in patient uncontrolled by drugs, those with recurrent strictures and in young patient unwilling for prolonged drug treatment.

  Surgery involves reduction of hiatus hernia if present; approximation of the crura around lower esophagus and some form of fundoplication

HIATUS HERNIA

- Abnormal protrusion of stomach through esophageal diaphragmatic hiatus into thorax.

Two types

1. Sliding hernia—stomach slides so that GE junction is in chest

2. Rolling or Paraesophageal hernia—though stomach rolls up, cardia is within abdominal cavity
   - CF: may be asymptomatic –heartburn—esophagitis and ulceration – bleed – anemia epigastric pain palpitation and hiccups

Invesigations: Barium meal and swallow OGD scopy X-ray chest reveal wide mediastinum and fluid level behind heart.

- Treatment: as per GERD

GASTRIC OUTLET OBSTRUCTION

- Commonly due to chronic duodenal ulcer with cicatrization
- Malignancy: stomach—antrum
- Malignancy of pancreas and lymphomas
- Crohn's disease of duodenum
- Adult hypertrophic pyloric stenosis
- Inflammation of adjacent organs with adhesions
- Gastroparesis
- Duodenal obstruction due to duodenal diverticula, duodinal atresia, annular pancreas, chronic duodenal ileus, superior mesenteric artery syndrome blockage by mesenteric lymphnodes.

PANCREATITIS

- Acute—after an attack of pancreatitis, organ returns to normalcy anatomically as well as functionally
- Chronic—associated with a permanent derangement of structure and function
- Gall stones and alcohol are important causes.

Causes of Acute Pancreatitis

- Non-traumatic (75%)

  Major factors:
  - Biliary disease(50%)
  - Alcohol (20–30%)

  Minor factors:
  - Viral—mumps, coxsackie
  - Drugs—steroids
  - Hyperparathyroidism
  - Hyperlipidaemia
  - Hypothermia
  - Scorpion sting
  - Carcinoma of pancreas
  - Previous polyarteritis and polyarteritis nodosa
- Traumatic (5%) operative, trauma, ERCP
- Idiopathic(20%).

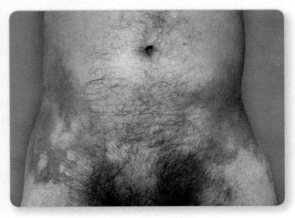

Figure 10.39: Grey Turner's sign

Pathophysiology

- Premature activation of pancreatic enzymes within duct system due to reflux of duodenal juice and or bile into pancreatic duct
- Intraductal activation of trypsin, chymotrypsin, phospholipase, catalase and elastase unleash chain of action—cell necrosis and change in microcirculation
- Rupture of duct leads to auto-digestion of gland
- Continuos release of activated proteolytic enzymes cause capillary permeability, protein exudation, retroperitoneal edema, peritoneal exudation
- Vasoactive kinins—kallikinin released
- Macrophages release cytokinins like tumor necrosing factor and interlukin
- Endotoxins are released.

General Effects

- Profound hypovolaemic shock due to altered capillary permeability and metabolic upsets due to cytokines
- Acute renal failure due to endotoxaemia, hypovolaemia and local intra vascular coagulation
- ARDS due to altered permeability of pulmonary capillaries
- Consumptive coagulopathy
- Altered liver function due to hepatocyte depression and/or obstruction of CBD by gall stone, pancreatic edema.

Clinical Features

- Agonizing constant epigastric pain radiating to back
- Marked retching, nausea and vomiting
- Exam reveals less features of tenderness, guarding and rigidity
- Cullen's sign

- Grey Turner's sign
- Obstructive jaundice
- Left sided pleural effusion

Diagnosis

- Key is high index of clinical suspicion and measurement of serum amylase
- Raised serum amylase at least three times the upper limit of normal(>1000 iu/ml)
- US and CT if needed.US reveals swelling of pancreas, peripancreatic collections and gall stones
- Diagnostic peritoneal lavage
- X-ray chest reveals left sided effusion
- X-ray abdomen—'sentinel loop' of jejunum and radio opaque gall stones.

Assessment of severity

- Glasgow system based on age, WBC count, blood glucose, serum urea, calcium, albumin, lactate dehydrogenase and serum aspartate aminotransferase—assessed within 48 hrs
- APACHE II score—C-reactive protein level
- Ronson's criteria—on admission and after 48hrs
- Edematous pancreatitis is usually mild and settles by conservative management
- Necrotising pancreatitis is severe; leads to complications and needs surgery—death

Treatment –conservative R regime

- **R**elive pain—Pethidine, Meperidine (no Morphine)
- **R**esuscitate—IV fluids and O_2
- **R**est the pancreas and bowel—Ryle's tube; nil oral
- **R**esist enzyme activity-? octerotide—somatostatin analogue
- **R**esist infection—antibiotics

- **R**epeated examination
- **R**epeated blood tests
- **R**espiratory support
- **R**enal output monitoring.

Endoscopic Treatment

- If gall stones are suspected to be the cause, endoscopic retrieval of such stones by basket or balloon after endoscopic sphincterotomy
- Patients with mild attack need no active therapy
- All patients with severe disease and cholangitis must undergo urgent ERCP and sphincterotomy.

Surgical Treatment

- Indications:
  1. uncertain diagnosis
  2. Patient fails to improve despite conservative management or deteriorates
  3. When gall stones are present
  4. When complications develop
- Laparotomy—Necrotic pancreatic and peripancreatic tissues removed from lesser sac by blunt dissection with finger and drains inserted. Gastrostomy or feeding jejunostomy if needed.

Complications

- Pancreatic pseudocyst
- Pancreatic abscess
- Pancreatic necrosis
- Progressive jaundice
- Persistent duodenal ileus
- GI bleeding
- Pancreatic ascites

- Roots of education are bitter but the fruit is sweet

Management Flow Chart: 1

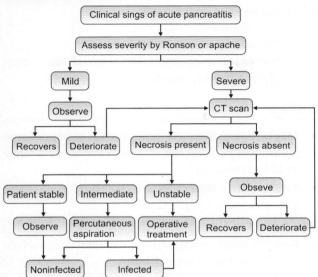

BLAST INJURIES

- Explosive pressure that accompanies bursting of bombs or shells produce rupturing of their cast and impart high velocity to resulting fragments
- Explosions manifest a complex blast wave with two components
  1. blast pressure wave with positive and negative phase
  2. Blast wind –movement of air
- Positive pressure last for milliseconds but rise up to 7000 kN/m² (tympanic membrane ruptures if more than 150 kN. Person is also affected by reflected pressure from surrounding. Blast wind disrupts the environment

- Middle ear, lungs, bowel affected
- Treatment
  - Resuscitation
  - Respiratory support
  - Regional management, be aware of PBRI—post blast respiratory insufficiency.

BURNS

- May be due to thermal injuries such as scalds or flame burns, electrical injuries, chemical injuries and rarely cold and radiation
- Most common organ affected is skin; but can also damage airway and lungs.

Assessment of Size

- Patient's hand correspond to 1% of total body surface area (TBSA) useful in small burns
- Large size to be assessed using Lund Browder chart rule if nine for first approximation.

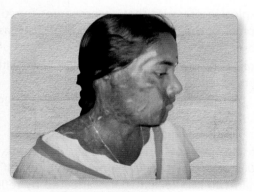

Figure 10.40: Post burns scar

Assessment of Depth

History is important—temperature, time and burnt material

- Superficial partial thickness—blistering with loss of epidermis .pinprick sensation normal
- Deep partial thickness—damage to deep reticular dermis. Reduced sensation
- Full thickness burns—hard ,leathery feel with no capillary return. No sensation(needle stuck deep without pain).

Treatment

- Fluid resuscitation plays a main role in treatment
- Burns > 10% TBSA in children and >15% TBSA in adults need iv fluids
- Parkland formula is widely used for calculating fluid replacement for first 24 hrs
- Total percentage of body surface area × weight in kg
- Half this volume to be given in first 8 hrs, second half to be given subsequent 10 hrs
- Ringer's lactate is the commonly used crystalloid—less expensive
- Human albumin solution(HAS) used in burns shock.

Management of Burn Wound

- Escharotomy , application of dressings with noncrystalline silver like silver sulphadiazine, mafinide acetate cream and cetrium nitrate
- Superficial wounds are treated by exposure
- Application of nonadhesive dressings with Vaseline impregnated dressings

---

- Knowledge is fire and it is antidote to fear

- Recently biological, synthetic and natural dressings like amniotic membranes are used.

ONYCHOCRYPTOSIS

- 'Ingrown' toe nails—pressure necrosis of nail wall and sulcus due to persistant contact with edge of nail plate leads to inflammation—suppuration—nil sulcus swells with exuberant granulation tissues
- Predisposing factors—shortly cut toe nail, soft pulp of debilitated persons, hyperhydrosis, ill fit or pointed shoes, subungual exostosis
- Treatment:
  Conservative—clean foot wear, proper nail trimming, thinning central part of nail by file
  Surgery—drain the pus by wedge excision of affected area-Watson-Cheyne operation nail bed ablation-Zadik's operation
- Onychogryphosis—overgrown toe nail—Ram horn toe.

PARONYCHIA

- Most common infection of hand caused by careless nail trimming or prick around nail fold skin, after initial inflammatory response pus trapped beside nail
- Incision and drainage with excision of outer quarter of nail
- Chronic paronychia is usually a fungal infection of occupation involving hand immersed in water
- Keep hands dry—anti fungal creams—if fails lay open nail bed

PULP SPACE INFECTION—FELON

- Terminal pulp space infection is the second most common infection of hand, follows minor injury—prick
- Terminal pulp space is a closed compartment and pressure increase due to infection compresses terminal artery—thrombosis—oesteomyeilitis (OM) of terminal phalanx
- Staphylo,strepto and Gm –ve organisms
- X-ray to rule out OM, pus culture and sensitivity
- Antibiotics +drainage of pus by oblique incision
- OM terminal phalanx needs amputation

CARCINOID SYNDROME

- Consists of periodic flushing, diarrhea, bronchoconstriction, wheezing and distinctive red-purple discoloration of face
- Right heart disease notably pulmonary stenosis may result –fatal
- 5HT and other biologically active amines are produced by gut carcinoids which are destroyed by liver; but if liver secondaries secrete these substances, they reach systemic circulation and produce carcinoid syndrome
- Detection of 5-hydroxy indol acetic acid in urine helps in diagnosis
- Primary tumor removed if possible
- Secondary excision of involved lobe,enucleation of the deposit or hepatic artery ligation / embolisation
- Symptomatic relief by blocking 5HT synthesis by alpha methyl dopa. Prevention of 5HT by somatostatin anologues.

DEEP VEIN THROMBOSIS (DVT)

- Occurs in 30% leg after major surgery. Starting point is a valve sinus in deep veins of calf usually asymptomatic, but early thrombus may get detached and emboli to lungs—fatal pulmonary embolism
- Risky patients—H/o previous DVT or embolism advanced age, malignancy, varicose veins, obese, major abdominal surgery, ortho surgery. (smokers have a low incidence!)
- Prophylaxis—low dose heparin 5000 units SC 8–12 hrly
- Duplex/Color Doppler is the key investigation
- If confined to calf, low risk of pulmonary embolism— Graded stockings and mobilisation
- Ileofemoral—highly risky—bed rest, anticoagulants— IV Heparin for a week followed by warfarin orally.

ADJUVANT CHEMOTHERAPY

- Aims to control the occult metastatic disease –given following surgery
- Different drugs act at specific points in cell cycle, hence a combination of drugs preferred—minimize side effects, reduces dosage
- Though given to destroy micro metastasis, patient sometimes may not have micro. Hence drugs given must have least toxicity and proven efficacy against the cancer treated.

NEOADJUVANT CHEMOTHERAPY

- Anterior Chemotherapy—Chemotherapy given prior to any surgical procedures in advance malignancies with a aim to downstage the malignancy.

HELICOBACTER PYLORI

- Gm negative, spiral, flagellate bacillus found in mucous lining human gastric epithelium and areas of gastric metaplasia in duodenum
- Infection common in peptic ulcer patients; evidence associates with gastric cancer
- Diagnosis: Invasive tests (following endoscopy). Rapid urease test(CLO test)—antral biopsy is inserted into a plastic slide with agar gel containing urea and pH indicator;if urease enzyme of *H. pylori* is present degradation of urea raise the pH—gel color changes to magenta from yellow

  Histology—staining of mucosa identifies

  Culture: in Columbia agar –prone for false negative Non-Invasive

  Tests: Breath test using isotope labeled CO_2

  Serology: Ig G antibodies against *H. Pylori* detected in the serum

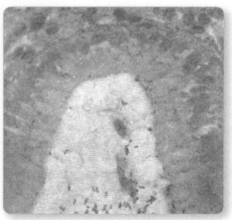

Figure 10.39: *Helicobacter pylori*

- Eradication:Triple drug regimen—Proton pump inhibitor metronidazole amoxycillin for 1 to 2 weeks.

GENE THERAPY

- Treatment by altering the genetic makeup of the patient. Recent exciting modality of treatment.
- Two methods—Germ cell therapy and Somatic cell therapy
- Germ cell therapy—insertion of a gene into a fertilized egg for correction of a genetic disease—passed into future generation
- Somatic cell therapy—insertion or manipulation of gene to treat a disease—not passed to germ cell line
- Vectors used—viral—retrovirus, adenovirus, herpes virus and vaccinia virus
  Non-viral systems—Liposome mediated DNA transfer DNA protein conjugates

Aims: 1. Repair or compensate for a defective gene

2. Enhance immune response directed towards tumor or pathogen
3. Kill tumor cells directly
4. Protect vulnerable cell population
5. Treatment of AIDS
6. Alter atherosclerosis

ORGAN TRANSPLANTATION

Aim: A transplanted organ must be accepted by its new host. Must remain capable of normal function at least enough function to support its new recipient.

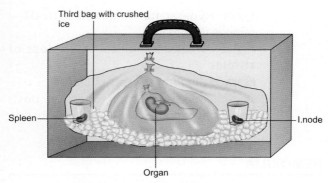

Third bag with crushed ice

Spleen

I.node

Organ

Figure 10.42: Mode of transport of organ

Harvest:
- May be from live related donor—parent or siblings
- Live unrelated donor
- Cadaver
    1. Must be of same blood group
    2. Tissue typing—donor lymphocytes versus recipient serum
    3. Determination of HLA antigen—done for all organ transplant—CDC (complement dependant cytotoxicity). Six antigen matches must be done for the recipient
- Post-transplantation care:
    - Immune suppressive treatment—drugs used single or in combination
    - Cyclosporine, steroids, azothiopurine, antibody (monoclonal and polyclonal) therapy
    - New-FK506 derived from fungal metobolite 100 times more potent than cyclosporine
- Rejection: Humoral and cell mediated

Types: Hyperacute—immediate in OT—remove the organ

Acute—weeks to month—high dose of steroids

Chronic—months to years

- Complications: Infection, rejection, post-transplant lymphoma 75%, skin malignancy, complications of steroids

HEMOBILIA

- Rare cause of acute or chronic blood loss from GIT leading to biliary colic and obstructive jaundice
- Causes: Traumatic liver and IVC injury leading to arteriobiliary communication Iatrogenic—difficult CBD exploration Gall stone disease—spontaneous or operated liver tumors and cholangio carcinoma communicating with bile ducts. Parasitic hepatobiliary infestations, vascular disorders
- In operated patients T tube indicates bleed
- Unoperated cases on suspicion do OGD scopy and ERCP
- US,CT,Selective angiogram to locate bleeding site
- Therapeutic embolisation or ligature of bleeding vessel
- Sandblom's triad—Melena, Jaundice, Pain

VESICAL CALCULUS

Stones in the urinary bladder
- Primary—originates in the kidney and passes to bladder where it enlarges—urine is sterile
- Secondary—forms within bladder in the presence of infection, bladder outlet obstruction or impaired bladder emptying

- Were widely prevalent due to poor protein intake—now diminished due to improvement in diet

Types
- Oxalate
- Uric acid
- Cystine
- Triple phosphate

Clinical features
- Male : female—8:1
- Frequency, strangury, terminal hematuria or acute retension of urine
- Strangury seen in patients with oxalate calculus
- Severe pain referred to tip of penis or labia majora at the end of micturition
- Symptoms of urinary tract infection (UTI)

Investigations
- Urine—reveals hematuria, pyuria and crystals of stone present (envelope-oxalate and hexagonal—cystine)
- X-ray KUB
- Cystoscopy—definite procedure both for diagnosis and treatment

Treatment
- Underlying cause to be treated
- BPH –prostatectomy should be done
- Endoscopy treatment is nowadays preferred
  Litholapaxy: stone crushed endoscopically; fragments evacuated by Ellick evacuator
- Percutaneous suprapubic litholapaxy—similar to percutaneous nephrolithotomy
- Open surgery
- Extra corporeal shock wave lithotripsy (ESWL)

CADAVERIC ORGAN TRANSPLANT

Donor: 1. Diagnosis compatible with brain death
2. Irreversible structural brain damage
3. Apnoeic coma

Unsuitable donors: 1. H/O malignancy except primary brain tumor and basal cell carcinoma (BCC) skin
2. Hepatitis B/C carrier
3. HIV positive
4. Major systemic sepsis
5. severe atherosclerosis.

- Multiorgan retrieval procedure—normally heart, lungs, liver, kidneys, pancreas,eyes,bone, and skin can be retrieved from same donor
- Thorough laparotomy to exclude any contraindications, e.g: undiagnosed bowel carcinoma
- Heart-lung removed en bloc after fully inflating lungs, stapling trachea and infusing cardioplegic lotion to cool and stop heart
- University of Wisconsin solution infused via portal canula for liver retrieval and storage. Liver is usually removed first en bloc with pancreas
- University of Wisconsin soln used in kidney also— removed last with samples of spleen and lymph node
- Donor iliac artery and vein are also taken and preserved
- Each organ is flushed again, placed in fresh perfusion soln; carried in two sterile plastic bags further placed in a bag with crushed ice within an insulated box for transport.

PRIMARY PERITONITIS

- Peritonitis is an inflammatory response of the peritoneal lining. Primary peritonitis is uncommon, accounts for 15% in childhood acute abdomen. common in young girls following ascent of pneumococcal or streptococcal infection from genital tract.
- *E. coli* is now the predominant causal organism which gain access through the gut wall or rarely blood borne spread from a distant focus.
- In adults spontaneous bacterial peritonitis SBP occur in patients with nephrotic syndrome, cirrhosis or CRF.
- CF: diffuse peritonitis with generalised abdominal tenderness and rigidity within 24 hours— fever,leucocytosis. Peritoneal fluid sample sent for C and S—gram staining.
- Treatment—antibiotic therapy is the mainstay. If needed laprotomy/laproscopy to exclude surgical cause if suggested by culture of enteric organism.

HIRSCHSPRUNG'S DISEASE

Definition: It is a congenital megacolon presenting with chronic constipation or large bowel destruction.

Pathology: Absence of ganglionic cells in the neural plexus of rectum and lower sigmoid colon due to failure of migration of neuroblasts into the gut from vagal nerve trunks.

Incidence: One in 4500 live births

- M > F
- 10% cases are associated with Down's Syndrome

Clinical Features: Neonates: delayed passage of meconium beyond first 24 hrs of life with abdominal distension and

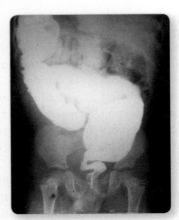

Figure 10.43: Hirschsprung's disease

bilious vomiting following feed – suggestive of large bowel obstruction.

- Gross abdominal distension, chronic constipation and failure to thrive.

Diagnosis: By full thickness rectal biopsy: histological demonstration of aganglionosis and hypertrophic nerve fibres.

- Anorectal manometry—absence of rectosphincteric inhibitory reflex
- Erect and supine X-ray of abdomen—distended loops of small and large intestine with fluid levels suggesting low intestinal obstruction
- Enema using water soluble contrast—defects in length and site of involved intestine

Treatment: Depends on age, length of involved segment, severity of symptoms and presence of enterocolitis.

- In neonates presenting with intestinal destruction or enterocolitis an initial colostomy is done
- In a child or adult with constipation alone—repeated enemas or rectal saline washouts to evacuate dilated intestine

Choice of surgery depend on length of involved segment.

Short Segment Disease

- Definitive surgery preceeds. Temporary colostomy for feed months to allow proximal distended colon to return to normal caliber
- In a neonate—definitive surgery deferred until child is 10 kg wt, 10 months to 1 year old

Surgical Procedures

- Duhamel operation: Excision of aganaglionic segment down to level of peritoneal reflexion and colorectal anastamosis
- Soave and Parks Coloanal anastamosis: Mucosectomy of the upper anal canal and rectum and coloanal anastamosis either directly or by stapling
- Swensens Procedure.

HYPERPARATHYROIDISM

- Primary—unstimulated and inappropriately high parathyroid hormone secretion for the concentration of plasma ionized calcium.due to adenoma or hyperplasia; rarely carcinomic
- Secondary—associated with chronic renal failure or malabsorption syndrome. All four glands are involved. Stimulus is chronic hypercalcemia
- Tertiary—further stage with autonomy;parathyroids no longer respond to physiological stimuli

Clinical Features

- Commoner in women
- Age 20 to 60 years
- Asymptomatic
- 'Bones, stones, abdominal groans and psychic moans'
- Only 50% suffer from any of these

Bone Diseases

- Generalised decalcification of skeleton as osteitis fibrosa cystica, single or multiple cysts or pseudo tumors of any bone
- Latter affects jaw bones
- Early radiological changes appear in skull bones and phalanges
- Mis diagnosed as rheumatic

Renal Stones

- Suspect in every patient with renal tract stone or nephrocalcinosis and even in cases of renal colic with no evidence of stone

Psychiatric Cases

- Not uncommon
- Tiredness, restlessness
- Personality changes make them labelled as 'neurotic and menopausal

Clinical Features

- Corneal calcification
- Band keratopathy
- Conjunctival calcification
- Hypertension
- Palpable adenoma neck seldom

Investigations
- Elevated serum calcium
- Diminished serum phosporus
- Increased excretion of urinary calcium
- Elevation of aerum alkaline phosphatase
- Elevation of parathormone

Differencial Diagnosis
- Secondary cancer in bone (breast, bronchus, prostate, kidney and thyroid)
- Carcinoma of endocrine secretion (bronchus,kidney and ovary)
- Multiple myeloma
- Vitamin D intoxication
- Sarcoidosis
- Thyrotoxicosis
- Immobilisation
- Medication—thiazide diuretics,lithium

Treatment
- Surgical removal of overactive gland/s
- Plastic and Reconstructive Surgery
- Keloid
- Split Thickness Skin Graft
- Cleft lip
- Cleft Palate
- Pedicle graft

SOLITARY RECTAL ULCER

- Anterior ulcer in the low rectum
- Rare condition difficult to treat effectively because there is a psychological overlay 20–40 years professional men or women
- Associated with introspective and anxious personality.

Differential diagnosis

1. Rectal carcinoma
2. Inflammatory bowel disease (Crohn's)
   Biopsy shows submucus fibrosis features with hypertrophy of muscularis mucosa and overlying ulceration.

Pathology

- Chronic straining due to constipation due to combination of internal intussusception or anterior rectal wall prolapsed and increase in intrarectal pressure.

Treatment

- Stool softeners
- Psychiatric help
- Better avoid surgery—abdominal rectopexy and rarely rectal excision.

SPLIT THICKNESS SKIN GRAFT (THIERSCH'S GRAFT)

- Taken with a special guarded free hand knife or an electrical dermatome
- Donor site heals with 2–3 weeks
- They can be expanded by meshing
- Thinner graft, better take up
- Used to cover wounds after acute trauma, granulating areas, burns and large defects.

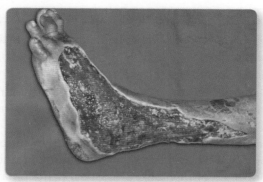

Figure 10.44: Raw area

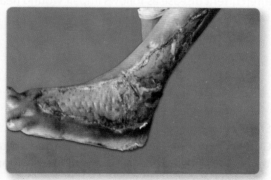

Figure 10.45: After SSG

FULL THICKNESS GRAFT

- Involves removal of full thickness of skin
- The donor defect has to be sutured or grafted
- Strong donot shrink but needs well vascularised bed to survive
- Commonly used in reconstructive surgery to cover the full defects of the palm and lower eyelid.

FACTORS AFFECTING WOUND HEALING

- Site of the wound and its orientation relative to tissue tension lines
- Good blood supply promotes healing
- General factors—age, presence of intercurrent infection, nutritional status and cardio-respiratory disease
- Local factors—bacterial contamination, antibiotic prophylaxis, aseptic technique degree of trauma, presence of devitalized tisssues, hematoma and foreign body
- Intercurrent disease as follows impair wound healing
  - Malnutrition
  - Diabetes mellitus
  - Hemorrhagic diathesis
  - Hypoxia
  - Corticosteroid therapy
  - Radiotherapy
- Surgical Technique
  Gentle handling, avoidance of undue trauma, meticulous haemostais accurate tissue positioning and approximation.

FLAPS

- Flaps bring their own blood supply to the new site
- Thicker and stonger than grafts
- Can be applied to avascular areas such as exposed bones, tendon or joints and mainly used for reconstruction of surgical defects and secondary reconstruction after trauma. For example:

TRAM (Tranversus abdominis myocutaneous flap)—for reconstruction of breast.
- LD—Lattisimus dorsi myocutaneous flap
- Berkamjian flap (PMMC)—Pectoralis major myocutaneous flap

TYPES OF HEMORRHAGE

- Primary
- Reactionary
- Secondary
- Primary refers to the bleeding at the time of injury or surgery
- Reactionary hemorrhage follow primary hemorrhage within 24 hours—mainly due to slippage of ligature, dislodgement of clot or cessation of reflux vasospasm—precipitated by:
  - Rise in BP and venous refilling following recovery from shock
  - Restlesness—coughing and straining—raise in venous
- Secondary hge occurs after 7–14 days, due to infection and sloughing of part of arterial wall. Precipitated by pressure of drainage tube, bone fragment, in infected area or cancer.
- Warning hge–bright red stains of dressings followed by sudden severe hge

AUTOTRANSFUSION

- The transfusion of patient's blood to self
- Used in three basic forms
  - Predeposit autologous blood donation
  - Preoperative isouaremic hemodilution

- Peroperative blood salvage
- Preoperative donation—blood withdrawn from fit patients awaiting elective surgery, 35–42 days prior. Upto 5 units. Prior to transfusion testing similar to allogenic donation
- Isovolumic dilution—upto 1.5 L of blood withdrawn into anticoagulant prior induction of anesthesia and replaced by saline. This blood is reinfused during surgery or in postop.
- Cell salvage—blood collected from operation site during surgery or by use of collection devices attached to surgical drains. Blood is processed by a cell salvage machine, where it is anticoagulated, cells are washed then returned to the patient. This procedure is contraindicated in malignancy and sepsis.

FRESH BLOOD COMPONENTS

- Whole blood
- RBC in additive solution
- Platelets
- Fresh frozen plasma (FFP)
- Cryoprecipitate

Plasma fractions

- Human albumin
- Prothrombin complex concentrates – II, IX and X may also contain factor VII
- Immunoglobulin preparations (90% Ig G)

UNIVERSAL PRECAUTIONS

HIV

- Prevention of needle stick injuries
- Use of gloves and gown

- Use of mask and eye covering
- Use of individual ventilation devices when need for resuscitation arises

Universal Precautions is Recommanded

- Blood, semen, vaginal secretions Amniotic fluid
- CSF
- Pericardial/peritoneal/pleural fluid
- Synovial fluid

Universal Precaution is not Recommended

- Feces
- Nasal secretion
- Sputum
- Sweat
- Tears
- Urine
- Vomitus

  Provided all these above are not blood stained

ACUTE APPENDICITIS

Acute inflammation of vermiform appendix

Clinical Features

- Pain abdomen –

  Classically starts as the periumbilical colic – mild to severe. It represents visceral pain due to appendiceal obstruction. Periumbilical location reflects the embryonic origin of appendix as a midline midgut structure. After several hours shifts to right iliac fossa – parietal peritonitis. Sharply located somatic pain
- Anorexia invariable with nausea
- Vomiting rarely a prominent feature
- Low grade temperature. Fever and tachycardia are not early signs of appendicitis.

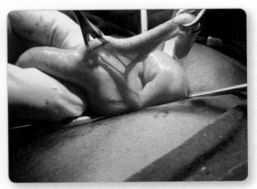

Figure 10.46: Appendicitis

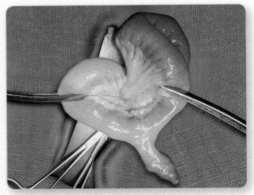

Figure 10.47: Meckel's Diverticulum

Important Signs in Appendicitis

- Tenderness in McBurney's point.
- Dunphy's sign (cough sign)—pain while coughing
- Murphy's triad—tenderness, pain, vomiting
- Hyperesthesia in RIF –> Murphy's syndrome

- Rowsing's sign—palpation of LIF result in pain in the RIF
- Blumberg's sign—rebound tenderness in RIF—sign of peritonitis
- Psoas sign—pain elicited by extending hip with knee in full extension
- Obturator sign—pain on flexion and internal rotation of the hip.

Pathology

- Obstructed appendix—accumulation of secretions—distension—necrosis of the mucosa
- Translocation of gut bacteria across the wall
- May resolve spontaneously or progress to gangrene and perforation as continuing obstruction impair blood supply
- Before frank perforation, bacteria migrate to peritoneal cavity—inflame parietal peritoneum
- Localized infection—appendicular mass or abscess
- Else—generalized peritonitis (more common in children, infants as omentum is not fully developed and localisation of infection is less effective).

Differential Diagnosis

Conditions that require surgery
- Perforated peptic ulcer
- Perforated carcinama of right colon
- Meckel's diverticulam
- Ectopic pregnancy
- Ovarian torsion
- Perforation of right colonic diverticulum

Conditions that do not require surgery

- PID
- Mittelschmertz
- Mesentric adenitis
- Viral gastroenteritis
- Typhoid
- Acute Crohn's ileus

Investigations

- Diagnosis is essentially clinical—repeated clinical examination
- Abdominal ultrasound—high resolution linear array transducer preferred-
  - Noncompressible appendix
  - Surrounded by hypoechoic area
  - Thickened wall of more than 2 mm in diameter
  - Maximum diameter exceeds 6 mm
  - Probe tenderness

  US excludes gynecological conditions and ureteric calculus
- Polymorphonuclear leucocytosis
  - 11000–17000 cells/mm^3
  - If more than 20000—perforation of appendix or other diagnosis
- Plain X-ray abdomen
  - Fecolith in 10% of cases
  - Localized ileus—distended small bowel loops
  - Obliteration of psoas border and free gas in late appendicitis
- Barium enema—done in children if diagnosis is uncertain
  - Spasm of terminal ileum or cecum

- External compression of cecum
- Non filling or partly filled appendix
- Pregnancy tests—to exclude ruptured ectopic
- Urine examination—may show pus or red cells if inflamed appendix is near urinary tract
- Laparoscopy
- CT and MRI
- CT features
  Pericecal inflammation signs, increase in density, thickened appendix, pericecal collection of fluid, pericolic adenopathy

Investigations to Improve the Diagnostic Accuracy

- Spiral CT scan with rectal contrast—more accurate than USG
- Thin cuts through the area of appendix
- Failure to fill the appendix by the contrast
- Mass effect in appendicular abscess
- Dirty fat sign, thickened mesoappendix, arrow head sign.

Treatment: Appendicectomy—surgical removal of appendix before gangrene or perforation

- Open method or laparoscopy
- Preoperative resuscitation required in the presence of generalised peritonitis—metronidazole and broad spectrum antibiotic cephalosporin

Various Incisions and Procedures

- Grid iron incision at the McBurney's point
- Rutherford Morrison's muscle cutting incision
- Lower right paramedian
- Lanz incision

Complications of Appendicitis

- Perforation
- Gangrene
- Pelvic abscess and intra abdominal abscess
- Portal vein thrombophlebitis-hepatic abscess

Appendiceal Mass and Abscess

- Keep D/D of Crohn's disease in mind
- Increasing pyrexia, pain and tenderness point to loculated pus – Appendicular abscess
- Abscess behind caecum and terminal ileum produce psoas spasm
- US and CT—helpful
- Appendix mass—conservative management
- Appendicular abscess—extraperitoneal drainage; if possible, Appendicectomy

Conservative Management

- **Oschner – Sherren** regime
    - Nil orally
    - Ryle's tube aspiration
    - IV fluids
    - Antibiotics

Stop and Proceed to Surgery if

- Rise in pulse rate
- Evidence of peritonitis
- Increasing / spreading abdominal pain
- Increase in the size of the mass as marked by skin pencil
- Vomiting / copius gastric aspirate

Normal Appendix Found at Surgery

- Exclude other pathologies
    - Mesenteric adenitis—yellow peritoneal fluid

- – Perforated peptic ulcer—bile stained fluid
- – Perforated colon—fecal fluid
- – Ischemic bowel—bloody fluid
- – Ectopic gestation—free blood
- Exclude Meckel's diverticulam and Crohn's disease and terminal ileitis
- Examine both ovaries and Fallopian tubes and sigmoid colon
- Even no other pathology is found—*do Appendicectomy* to avoid confusion later due to the scar in RIF.

ACUTE CHOLECYSTITIS

- Acute inflammation of gall bladder—majority associated with gall stones and results from obstruction of gall bladder outflow

Clinical Features

- Patient looks unwell, has pyrexia with severe right hypochondrial pain
- Pain radiates to subscapular area (Boas sign) and rarely to right shoulder

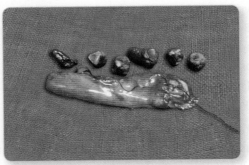

Figure 10.48: Calculous cholecystitis

- Tachycardia, nausea, vomiting
- Abdominal tenderness and rigidity
- Murphy's sign
- Palpable mass due to wrapped omentum

Investigations

- Blood count—leucocytosis
- Liver function tests—mild derangement
  Serum bilirubin—5 mg/dL in 20% cases due to choledochal inflammation values more than 5 mg/dL imply CBD stones
- Serum amylase—to determine associated pancreatic inflammation
- X-ray chest—to rule out pneumonia
- Electrocardiogram—to rule out cardiac cause
- Urine microscopy and culture—to rule out renal disease

Imaging Studies

Ultrasound Study

- First line of investigation
- Sensitivity is 90%
- Hyperechoeic with acoustic shadow
- GB wall thickening and edema more than 5 mm
- Pericholecystic fluid
- Positive sonographic Murphy's sign
- Biliary sludge

Plain X-ray Abdomen

- 10% stones—radio opaque
- Gas in the GB Wall [emphysematous cholecystitis]
- Gall stone ileus [Rigler's triad-gas in GB, small bowel dilatation and stone in RIF]

- Mercedes Benz Sign
- Gas in biliary tree (bilioenteric fistula)

Radio Nucleotide Scanning

- The diagnostic tool of choice in acute cholecystitis
- Di-isopropyl derivatives of technetium 99m-HIDA and IODIDA are used.
- 95% accurate, reflects the biliary function
- US and radionucleotide scanning are complementary
- CT
- ERCP
- MRCP

Differential Diagnosis

Common Conditions

- Appendicitis
- Perforated peptic ulcer
- Acute pancreatitis

Other Conditions

- Acute pyelonephritis of right kidney
- Myocardial infarction
- Right lower lobe pneumonia

Treatment

Concepts of surgical intervention—*cholecystectomy*
Though many surgeons favor conservative management, nowadays surgeons prefer early surgery in the absence of any medical contraindications within 5 to 7 days. But usually surgery is done after 6 weeks (till subsidence of inflammation).

Conservative Line of Management

1. Nasogastric aspiration and intravenous fluid administration
2. Administration of analgesics
3. Administration of antibiotics
4. Subsequent management after the inflammation subsides
   – Nasogastric tube removed
   – Oral fluids followed by fat-free diet
   – Ultrasound to ensure no complications and normal CBD

Emergency Surgery is Indicated

- Progression of disease
- Failure to improve within 24 hrs of treatment
- Detection of gas in GB and biliary tree
- Established generalized peritonitis
- Development of intestinal obstruction

ACALCULOUS CHOLECYSTITIS

- Acute and chronic cholecystitis in the absence of stones
- Clinical features similar to calculus cholecystitis
- Common in critically ill patients undergone major surgery, trauma and burns
- Mortality high as diagnosis is often missed
- Treatment—emergency cholecystectomy; if not cholecystostomy.

ACUTE INTESTINAL OBSTRUCTION

- Any form of impedance to the normal passage of bowel contents through small or large intestine
- Obstruction may be mechanical or functional

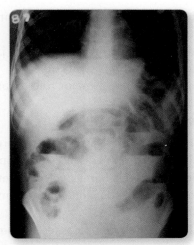

Figure 10.49: Multiple fluid levels—intestinal obstruction

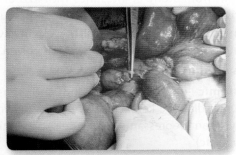

Figure 10.50: Congenital band—intestinal obstruction

Mechanical obstruction is due to a physical blocking of the lumen of the Intestine

- Extrinsic , intrinsic or from within lumen
- **Small bowel**—adhesions are the commonest cause 60%, hernias 20%, malignancy10%

- **Large bowel**—malignancy most common 65%, diverticular disease 10%, volvulus 5%
- Adhesions are due to a reduction in peritoneal plasminogen activating activity (PAA)
- In India volvulus play a major role in large bowel obstruction.

Causes of Mechanical Obstruction

- **Intrinsic**—congenital atresia, strictures due to tuberculosis and Crohn's disease and neoplasms
- **Extrinsic**—adhesions, hernia, volvulus, intussusceptions, congenital bands , inflammatory masses and neoplasms
- **Luminal**—FB, gall stones, parasites and bezoars.

Functional Obstruction

- Results from atony of intestines with loss of normal peristalsis, in the absence of a mechanical cause
- Termed as paralytic ileus if small bowel is involved and pseudo-obstruction if large bowel is involved.

Causes of Functional Obstruction

- **Systemic**—metabolic, drug induced, sepsis and trauma(diabetic ketoacidosis, uremia, dehydration, tricyclic antidepressants, GA, acute pancreatitis, head injury, etc)
- **Local**—affecting bowel motility(-peritonitis, infections, strongyloides and postoperative ileus).

CLINICAL FEATURES AND MANAGEMENT

General Principles

- The bowel proximal to the obstruction dilates— accumulation of gas and fluid—loss of water and

electrolytes into the bowel lumen—patient shows signs of dehydration
- Dilatation activates stretch receptors resulting in reflex contraction of smooth muscle—colicky pain and distension of abdomen
- If obstruction is not overcome, the bowel activity ceases resulting in atony unless strangulation or perforation intervenes.

Small Bowel Obstruction

- Colicky pain and vomiting are the early features
- Constipation is a late feature
- In distal small bowel obstruction onset is insidious: vomiting may become feculant.
- Always examine hernial orifices
- PR may reveal faecal impaction or rectal tumor, diverticula or malignant deposits
- Suspect strangulation if
  - Abdominal tenderness on palpation
  - Tachycardia
  - Pyrexia
  - Colicky pain replaced by continuous dull ache or is associated with a background of constant pain
  - Plain X-ray abdomen—small bowel distension (> 2.5 cm) confirms diagnosis.
- If strangulation is suspected emergency surgery after resuscitation
- Strangulated bowel is blue or black, lustreless, absence of peristaltic activity and no arterial pulsation in adjacent mesentery
- Resection of that loop with end-to-end anastomosis or exteriorization of divided ends of intestine

- If no suspicion of strangulation
  - Nasogastric decompression
  - IV fluid replacement
  - Electrolyte monitoring and correction.

Large Bowel Obstruction

- Though 3–4 times less common than small bowel obstruction , it requires surgical intervention more commonly
- Malignancy is most common cause, almost equal incidence of sigmoid volvulus in India
- Most patients are constipated with laxative abuse
- Abdominal distension and constipation are early features
- Colicky painless marked—vomiting very late
- PR mandatory—presence of blood and mucous in the glove suggest distal neoplasm
- Sigmoidoscopy—visualise obstructing lesion and also helps to decompress sigmoid volvulus
- Plain X-ray abdomen and CT if needed
- Full resuscitation followed by laparotomy.
- Surgery in accordance to the cause made out.

CLOSED LOOP OBSTRUCTION

- This occurs when the bowel is obstructed at both the proximal and distal points.
- Unlike non-strangulating obstruction no early distension of proximal bowel
- Imminent gangrene of the strangulated segment leads to retrograde thrombosis of the mesenteric vein resulting in distension on both sides of strangulated segments

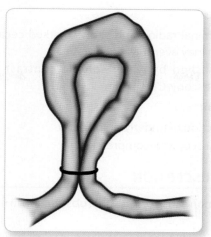

Figure 10.51: Closed loop obstruction

- Classic form seen in malignant stricture of right colon with the competent ileocecal valve
- Unrelieved, this results in necrosis and perforation

PSEUDO-OBSTRUCTION

- Colonic obstruction with no mechanical cause
- May be acute or chronic
- Acute colonic pseudo-obstruction is known as **Ogilvie's syndrome**

Predisposing Causes

Systemic: Metabolic, drug induced, sepsis and trauma (diabetic ketoacidosis, uremia, dehydration, tricyclic antidepressants, GA. Acute pancreatitis, head injury, etc)

Local: Affecting bowel motility(-peritonitis, infections, strongyloides and postoperative ileus)

Diagnosis

- Abdominal radiograph shows marked cecal dilation which may eventually perforate
- Established by water soluble contrast enema / colonoscopy/CT

Treatment

- Correction of underlying disorder
- Colonoscopic decompression.

INTUSSUSCEPTION

- Common cause of intestinal obstruction in first year of life
- Terminal ileum peristalsed into the cecum and ascending colon (ileocolic intussusception)
- Commonly occurs following viral illness—enlargement of Peyer's patches in terminal ileum which becomes lead point(apex)
- In older children small bowel polyps, tumors, hamartomas as in Henoch-Schonlein purpura and Meckel's diverticulum act as lead points (ileocolic, ileoileal or ileoileocolic)

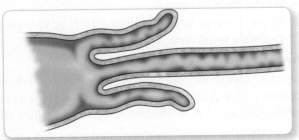

Figure 10.52: Ileocolic intussusception

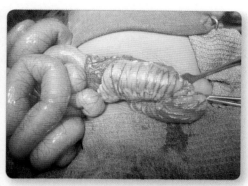

Figure 10.53: Intussusception

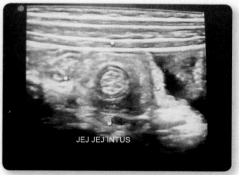

JEJ JEJ INTUS

Figure 10.54: Intussusception—target sign

Clinical Features

- Screaming attacks with pallor and drawing up of knees
- Anorexia and vomiting
- Normal pattern of stooling disrupted
- Distended ,tender abdomen—passing "*Red currant jelly*" stools
- Dehydration, infant drowsy and unrousable

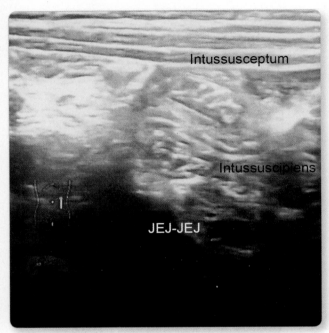

Figure 10.56: Intussusception USG

- Abdominal examination reveals empty right iliac fossa with a sausage shaped mass concave towards umbilicus in the right upper quadrant- *'Sign de dance'*.
- Abdominal ultrasound to confirm diagnosis
- Transverse scanning reveals '**Target sign**' (Rings of the target representing various layers of the bowel wall)

Management

- Correction of dehydration
- Pneumatic reduction of intussusception using an air enema under X-ray screening
- Failure to reduce in this way requires laparotomy and reduction or resection of the affected bowel.

PERFORATED PEPTIC ULCER

More common in duodenal ulcer than gastric ulcer (bleeding more in gastric in contrast)

Pathogenesis

- Perforation occurs through floor due to impaired blood supply— endarteritis
- **Duodenal ulcer** perforates from anterior wall 92%
- Upto 50% no previous ulcer symptoms
- **Gastric ulcer** perforates mostly from anterior or anterosuperior region of lesser curvature
- Strong association with NSAID (nonsteroidal anti-inflammatory drug) use.

Clinical features

- May be h/o peptic ulcer, NSAID intake
- Usually insidious with increasing pain abdomen
- 5% present with sudden, severe unremitting abdominal pain, tachycardia and ileus.

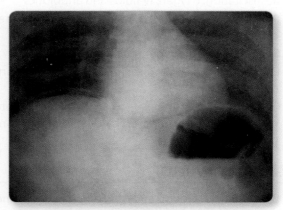

Figure 10.56: Air under diaphragm - pneumoperitoneum

- Range of symptoms depend on intra-abdominal course
- Irritant stomach contents may cause shoulder tip pain—sub diaphragmatic irritation
- Vomiting may occur. Abdomen does not move freely with respiration
- **O/E** – Abdominal guarding and rebound tenderness
  - Involuntary board like rigidity
  - Absence of liver dullness
  - Absence of bowel sounds
  - Late cases present with fulminant peritonitis

Diagnosis

- Erect X-ray chest- free air under right dome of diaphragm (fundus air shadow may be seen normally under left dome)
- If patient is sick, left lateral decubitus X-ray helpful
- Moderate hyperamylasemia
- If needed Gastrograffin (water soluble contrast) study.

Management

- Resuscitation, oxygen, IV fluids and antibiotics
- Adequate analgesics, anti emetics, urinary catheterisation
- **Surgery**—thorough peritoneal lavage
- DU perforation—simple closure of perforation—omental patch
- Gastric ulcer perforation—as 15% prove ultimately malignant , biopsy followed by closure or excision of ulcer.

SIGMOID VOLVULUS

- Due to a twist around a narrow origin in the sigmoid mesentery

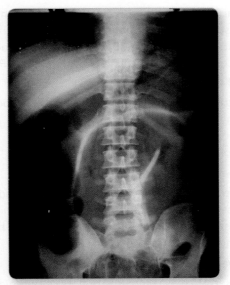

Figure 10.57: Sigmoid volvulus—Plain X-ray abdomen

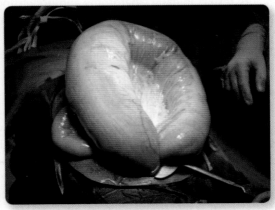

Figure 10.58: Sigmoid volvulus

- An acquired condition in elderly patients with chronic constipation
- Most common cause of large bowel obstruction in places with high level of dietary fibre—India, Pakistan.

Clinical Presentation

- Features of bowel obstruction with lower abdominal pain
- Abdominal distension, nausea, vomiting
- Absolute constipation.

Plain X-ray

- *Coffee bean sign*—Y shaped shadow surrounded by a grossly distended colon arising out of pelvis
- Water soluble contrast show characteristic `beaking' at the site of twist.

Treatment

- Conservative by using rigid or flexible sigmoidoscope by reduction and deflation
- Failure results in early laparotomy and untwisting of the loop and fixation of loop to posterior abdominal wall
- If suspicion of strangulation or gangrene—emergency laparotomy and resection.

MUCOCELE OF GALLBLADDER

- Obstruction to neck of gallbladder by stone with sterile contents bile is absorbed—replaced by mucus secretion by GB epithelium palpable GB of enormous size
- Mucocele can also occur in malignancy which occludes the cystic duct like cholangiocarcinoma
- Pus replacement–Empyema
- R_x Cholecystectomy.

Case Presentation

Presentation of long case must be written as a complete case sheet with complete diagnosis, whenever needed differential diagnosis and management consisting of necessary investigations and treatment.

Short cases needs no case sheet but student must do proper local examination and present properly.

The pattern of case presentation is as follows:

1. Common data—name, age, sex, occupation and place
2. Chief complaints—in the patient's own words, in the chronological order
3. History of present illness—onset, duration and progression of symptoms
4. History suggestive of relevant etiological factors including negative history
5. Past history—routinely about hypertension, diabetic status and exposure to TB illness.
   Any previous surgery, STD exposure and any other ailments
6. Personal history—diet, addiction to alcohol, tobacco, etc.
7. Family history
8. Treatment history
9. General examination
10. Local examination

11. Systemic examination
12. Diagnosis
13. Investigations
14. Treatment—pertaining to the given case.

Typical Case Sheets

INGUINAL HERNIA

Mr/Mrs............................... aged.......... hails from.......
occupation as...........

Complains of swelling in the inguinal region that appears on straining for the past .... months.

H/O Present Illness

About the appearance of swelling and modality of reduction—by the patient or automatically when patient lies down associated with gurgling noise or not

Past History

- Any history of chronic cough, difficulty in passing motion, micturition
- Past history of exposure to STD—(remember gonococcal urethritis leads to stricture of urethra)
- Any previous surgery for hernia(recurrence) abdominal surgery (appendicectomy by Rutherford Morrison's muscle cutting incision may lead to direct hernia due to injury to ileo hypogastric nerve).

Local Examination

- Examine the patient on erect as well as lying down position and mention this in the case sheet. Inspection—describe the shape, size and extent of the swelling and describe the expansile cough impulse. Palpation—warmth, tenderness consistency

- Feel for the expansile cough impulse at the root of scrotum
- Getting above is not possible in inguinoscrotal swellings
- Assess the mode of reduction
- Do the deep ring occlusion test, finger invagination test external ring and Zieman's method of palpation
- Examine other inguinal region, scrotum and penis
- Abdomen—tone of muscles, Malgaigne bulges, presence of lump/ free fluids
- RS. CVS and other systems
- Diagnosis: type, side, complete or incomplete, complicated or not.

VARICOSE VEINS

- Name, age, sex, place of the patient with his Occupation
- Complains of—unsightly swelling—dull aching pain—pigmentation, swelling and ulcer of leg/ankle
- Past history of thrombophlibitis, females—pregnancy associated.

Clinical Examination

- Done both in standing and lying down positions
- Compare both lower limbs, remember localized gijantism in AV malformations
- Look for skin pigmentations, lipodermosclerosis, ulcer
- Look at the attitude of foot(for equinous deformity)
- Describe cough impulse—morrisis cough impulse seen at saphenofemoral junction
- Describe the varicose vein.

Palpation

- Warmth, tenderness
- Fegan's method of palpation—look out for blow outs
- Moses test and Homan's test for deep vein status
- Feel for the cough impulse
- Special tests: 1. Trendelenburg test
                2. Multiple tourniquet test
                3. Modified Perthe's test.

Percussion

- Schwartz—tap a single column of blood
- Auscultation—look for continous machinery murmur in A-V Fistula
- *Diagnosis:* Long or short saphenous vein varicosity with sapheno-femoral incompetence or saphenopopliteal incompetence—with or without perforator incompetence—with or without complication.

THYROID SWELLING

Name.........sex...aged....occupation ....place from which hails

- C/o swelling neck since.........
- H/o present illness: Swelling when noted——progression—any increase or decrease in size
- H/o pain, discomfort on swallowing
- H/o pressure effect
- H/o symptoms of thyrotoxicosis—
  CNS: Irritability, insomnia, tremours
  CVS: Palpitations, dyspnea on exertion
- Metabolic and GIT: Loss of weight despite good appetite, diarrhea, poor heat tolerance

- Oligomenorrhea, amenorrhea
- H/o hypothyroidism— weight gain, slow speech and action, loss of hair, fatigue, constipation—menorrhagia
- Eye symptoms: Starring eye, difficulty in closing eyes (exophthalmos) double vision due to muscle weakness (ophthalmoplegia), congestion of conjunctiva (chemosis)
- Family H/o—similar swellings—endemic goitre, dyshormonogenesis, autoimmune conditions like Grave's, Hashimotos thyroiditis

General Exam
- Mental status to be assessed in addition to routine
- Look for eye signs and tremors.

Local Examination
Inspection: Describe the swelling and say about movement on deglutition—whether lower border seen or not; in case of solitary swellings look for movement on protrution of tongue—describe the exterior—position of trachea—look for any other swelling in the neck.

Palpation
- Warmth, tenderness—consistency, movement on deglution—
- Assess the plane—skin pinchable—becomes less prominent on stretching investing layer of deep cervical fascia—less prominent on contracting infrahyoid strap muscles—moves on deglution as it is attached to trachea by Berry's ligaments
- Feel for thrill at upper pole
- Feel the common carotid pulsation just below the upper border of thyroid cartilage in front of

sternomastoid on the transverse process of C6 Position of trachea

- Feel for any other swelling in the neck
- Auscultation—if thrill is present
- Percussion—mediastinum to be percussed when there is retrosternal extension
- Examine CVS, CNS
- Diagnosis: Nature—diffuse or multinodular—solitary
- Toxic or nontoxic—malignant or nonmalignant.

CASE OF TAO

- A male aged….., occupation and place
- C/o pain leg while walking, ulcer—gangrene toe
- Present Illness: onset and progression of complaints
- Personal H/o—diet, alcohol intake
- Smoking—beedi or cigar …..packets per day since….. years

Local Examination

- Comparison of both lower limbs
- Description of gangreneous area in detail
- Mark of demarcation present
- Pulse chart—both lower limbs and upper limbs
- Dorsalis pedis, posterior tibial, popliteal, femoral pulses
- Radial, brachial, axillary , superficial temporal pulses
- Other system: CVS, RS, CNS
- Diagnosis: a case of peripheral vascular disease—TAO
- Investigations and treatment.

ABDOMINAL LUMPS

- C/o lump abdomen or pain abdomen since………..

- H/o present illness—onset-progression
- Nature of pain—aggravating, relieving factors
- Associated with vomiting—hemetemesis, melena
- Loss of appetite, weight
- General examination: in cases c/o vomiting signs of dehydration to be noted.

Local Examination

Inspection

- Shape of abdomen, movement of areas during respiration, position of umbilicus, loin, groin, inguinal region, presence of visible peristalsis, state of abdominal wall are noted; left supraclavicular region examined
- In case of a visible lump the size, area occupied, movement with respiration written
- Head raising test or straight leg raising test are done. Intra-abdominal lump becomes less prominent.

Palpation

- Warmth and tenderness noted
- Lump measured, movement with respiration, intrinsic mobility assessed
- Patient put on knee-chest position and lump palpated—intraperitoneal lump falls forward, better palpated but retroperitoneal lump does not fall forward.

Percussion

- Lump arising from GI tract have impaired dullness and lump from solid organs like liver, spleen are dull

- Shifting dullness of free fluid seeked—Puddle sign for small amount of fluid—fluid thrill.

Auscultation
Other systems
Diagnosis
- Investigation and Treatment

A CASE OF GOO DUE TO CICATRIZED DUODENAL ULCER

- C/o burning sensation—pain abdomen—vomiting etc.
- H/o present illness: onset and progression of symptoms
- H/o ball rolling movements
- Details of vomiting—when it occurs, content of vomitus
- H/o hemetemesis, malena
- Past H/o periodicity of peptic ulcer pain
- Personal H/o—diet, alcohol and tobacco.

General Examination

- Look for signs of dehydration

Local Examination

- Succussion splash
- VGP
- Auscultopercussion for dilated stomach—greater curvature marked
- Other systems
- *Diagnosis:* A case of gastric outlet obstruction probably due to cicatrized duodenal ulcer.

CARCINOMA BREAST

C/o lump in the breast for………..

Discharge..pain…

H/O Present Illness

- Time of noticing the lump and progression
- Any change in nipple(recent retraction)
- Discharge—spontaneous or induced-color

Past History

- Similar episodes in past—availability of biopsy report (Atypical Epithelial Hyperplasia deserves special attension)
- OCP Intake in premenopausal women and HRT postmenopausal women.

Family History

- First degree relatives with carcinoma breast
- Menstrual history: Age of menarche, details of periods, whether menstruating or not-menopause age
- Marietal history: Age of marriage, first childbirth, number of children details of lactation.

Local Exam

- Compare both breasts, level of nipple
- Presence of lump—quadrant occupied
- Skin manifestations—tethering/dimpling, infiltration, peau' de orange, ulceration, carcinoma en cruissae any fullness in axilla, supraclavicular area

Palpation

- Lump better appreciated by palmar aspect of fingers—warmth and tenderness

- Consistency hard
- Mobility—moves along with breast tissue
- Upper outer lump—whether attached to pectorolis maj or not
- Lower outer lump—whether attached to serratus anterior or not
- Nipple and areola examined—for discharge and retraction
- Axillary nodes examined—size, shape, group, consistency and mobility made out
- Always examine normal breast and axilla(better early)
- Abdomen examined for evidence of organomegaly, free fluid and lump (Krukenberg tumour in premenopausal women)
- Respiratory system for evidence of effusion
- Areas of bony tenderness

Diagnosis

Carcinoma breast- involving ......

Clinical staging

TNM Staging

University Question Bank

SHORT NOTES

Disorders of Salivary Glands

1. Pleomorphic adenoma
2. Parotidectomy
3. Warthin's tumor
4. Sialogram
5. Frey's syndrome

Pharynx Larynx and Neck

1. Cystic hygroma
2. Cervical rib
3. Carotid body tumor
4. Branchial cyst
5. Dentigerous cyst

Burns

1. Electrical burns
2. Marjolin's ulcer
3. Surgical treatment of burns

Urology

1. Bladder diverticulum
2. Fournier's gangrene
3. Ureteric calculus
4. Polycystic kidney
5. Congenital hydrocele

6. Undescended testis
7. Priapism
8. ESWL
9. Causes of retention of urine
10. Vesical calculus
11. Wilm's tumor
12. Perinephric abscess
13. Varicocele
14. No scalpel vasectomy
15. Torsion of testis
16. Paraphimosis
17. Hypospadiasis
18. Encysted hydrocele
19. Complications of pelvic ring disruption

Hernia, Umbilicus and Abdominal wall

1. Incisional hernia
2. Femoral hernia
3. Encysted hydrocele of cord
5. Epigastric hernia

The Thyroid Gland and Thyroglossal Tract

1. Solitary nodule thyroid
2. Complications of thyroid surgery
3. Hypoparathyroidism
4. Hashimoto's thyroiditis
5. Thyroglossal cyst
6. Principles of management of thyrotoxicosis
7. Lingual thyroid
8. Postoperative complications of thyroid surgery
9. Principles of management of thyrotoxicosis

Parathyroid and Adrenal Gland

1.   Brown's tumor
2.   Cushing's syndrome
3.   Tetany

Cardiac surgery

1.   Empyema thoracis
2.   Intercostal drainage
3.   Cardiac tamponade
4.   CABG

Principles of Pediatric surgery

1.   Hirschsprung's disease
2.   Trachoesophagal fistula
3.   Meconium ileus
4.   Umbilical fistulae
5.   Umbilical hernia
6.   Umbilical adenoma

Elective Neurosurgery

1.   EDH
2.   Depressed fracture of skull
3.   Extradural hemorrhage
4.   Glasgow coma scale
5.   Subdural hematoma

Anesthesia and Pain Management

1.   Spinal anesthesia
2.   Cardiac arrest
3.   Muscle relaxants
4.   Epidural anesthesia
5.   Brachial plexus block

Transplantation

1.   Immunosuppressive therapy

Wound Infection

1. Hilton's Method of I and D
2. Carbuncle
3. Nosocomial infections
4. Cold abscess
5. Tuberculous lymphadenitis
6. Anthrax
7. Management of tetanus
8. Amebic liver abscess
9. Universal precaution
10. Gas gangrene
11. Postexposure prophylaxis.
12. Tetanus prophylaxis

Acute Life Support and Critical Care, Blood Transfusion and Blood Products

1. Septic shock
2. Neurogenic shock
3. Acid-base disturbance
4. Metabolic alkalosis
5. Metabolic acidosis
6. Hypokalemia
7. Cardiac tamponade
8. Rh factor
9. Complications of blood transfusion
10. Complication of massive blood transfusion
11. Autotransfusion
12. Blood product

The Peritoneum Omentum Mesentry and Retro Peritoneal Space

1. Tuberculous peritonitis
2. Koch's abdomen

Venous Disorder

1. Chronic venous ulcer
2. Complications of varicose veins
3. A-V fistula
4. Therapeutic embolisation
5. Venogram
6. Raynauds phenomenon
7. Hemangioma
8. DVT—of lower limb and its prevention
9. Prevention of DVT
10. Postphlebitis leg

The Breast

1. Cystosarcoma phylloides
2. Phylloides tumor
3. Nipple discharge
4. Antibioma
5. Breast abscess
5. Mammography
6. Fibroadenosis of breast
7. Paget's disease of breast
8. Retromammary abscess
9. TNM Classification of carcinoma breast
10. Etiological factors of carcinoma breast
11. Lymphatic drainage of breast

The Rectum

1. Piloinidal sinus
2. Fistulogram
3. Goodsall's rule
4. Hemorrhoids
5. Acute fissure-in-ano

6. Appendicular lump
7. Sigmoid volvulus
8. Colostomy
9. Management of prolapsed rectum
10. Carcinoid tumor of appendix
11. Rectal polyp
12. Pelvic abscess
13. Sigmoid volvulus
14. Solitary rectal ulcer
15. Colostomy
16. Ameboma
17. Paralytic ileus
18. Oschner–Sherron's regime

Cysts Ulcers and Sinuses

1. Lipoma
2. Melanoma
3. Pressure sores
4. Thyroglossal cyst
5. Hemangioma
6. Rodent ulcer
7. Branchial cyst
8. Premalignant conditions of skin
9. Malignant melanoma
10. Epidermoid cyst
11. FNAC
12. Trophic ulcer
13. Marjolin's ulcer
14. Paronychia
15. Dermoid cyst
16. Classification of cyst

17. Actinomycosis
18. Fournier's gangrene
19. Clinical staging of Hodgkin's lymphoma

Oral and Oropharyngeal Cancer

1. Cleft lip
2. Cleft palate
3. Ranula
4. Carcinoma cheek
5. Cancrum oris
6. Leukoplakia
7. Dentigerous cyst
8. Adamantinoma
9. Premalignant oral lesions
10. Dental cyst

Pancreas, Liver and Gall Bladder and Bile Duct

1. Pseudocyst of pancreas
2. Pancreatic fistula
3. Hydatid liver disease
4. Amebic liver abscess
5. Hyadatid cyst
6. Gaucher's disease
7. Budd-Chiari syndrome
8. Hemobilia
9. Etiopathogenesis of gall stones
10. Biliary colic
11. Charcot's triad

The Thorax

1. Hemangioma
2. A-V fistula

3. Tension pneumothorax
4. CABG
5. Hemopneumothorax
6. Pulmonary embolism
7. Pancoast tumor
8. Empyema necessitans
9. Intercostal drainage
10. Empyema thoracis

Esophagus, Stomach, Small Intestine

1. Achalsia cardia
2. Barret's esophagus
3. Tracheoesophageal fistula
4. Corrosive gastritis
5. *H. Pylori*
6. Acute dilatation of stomach
7. GOO
8. Intussusception
9. Mesentric cyst
10. Meconeum ileus
11. Peutz-Jeghers syndrome

The Spleen

1. Complications of splenectomy
2. Splenic trauma
3. Indications for splenectomy
4. Infarction of the spleen
5. Rupture of spleen management
6. Splenosis
7. Biological substances removed by spleen

Arterial Disorders

1. Raynaud's phenomenon
2. TAO

Vermiform Appendix

Acquired Immuno Deficiency Syndrome

1. Infection in AIDS

Day Surgery

1. Day care surgery

Basal Cell Carcinoma

1. Rodent ulcer
2. Frey's syndrome
3. BCC

Diagnostic and Interventional Radiology

1. FNAC
2. Nasogastric aspiration
3. IVU
4. Radio active isotopes
5. ERCP
6. DSA
7. OGD scopy
8. Venogram
9. CVP measurement
10. Sialogram
11. MRI
12. MRCP
13. PET scan
14. CT scan
15. USG

Miscellaneous

1. Needle stick injury
2. Horner's syndrome
3. Desmoid tumor
4. Collar stud abscess
5. Factors affecting wound healing
6. Scalpels used in surgery
7. ATLS—advanced trauma life

Nutrition

1. Complications of TPN
2. Parenteral nutrition

Principles of Laparoscopic surgery

1. Diagnostic laparoscopy
2. Advantages of minimal access surgery

Treatment-questions

1. Pelvic abscess
2. Therapeutic embolization
3. Immunosuppressive therapy
4. Triage
5. Prophylactic antibiotics in surgery

ESSAY

Thyroid

1. Classify thyroid carcinoma. Discuss etiology, clinical features, investigation and treatment of a 2 cm nodule in the right lobe of thyroid of a 40-year-old male patient proven on FNAC to be papillary carcinoma.
2. A 40-year-old female with thyroid enlargement—pulse rate 95/min.DD of management.

3. Clinical features of thyrotoxicosis and management of secondary thyrotoxicosis.

   Differential diagnosis of a solitary nodule of right lobe of thyroid in a 35-year-old female. Diagnosis and management of follicular carcinoma of thyroid.

4. A 30-year-old female comes to the hospital with clinically nontoxic solitary nodular goiter – discuss the differential diagnosis, relevant investigation and management of papillary carcinoma thyroid.

5. A 35-year-old lady comes to the hospital with swelling in the anterior aspect of neck which moves up with deglutition
   a. Enumerate the possible causes.
   b. How will you investigate the case?
   c. Write briefly about the management of thyrotoxicosis.

Breast

6. A 50-year-old female came to the OPD with painless hard lump in the right breast. Describe in detail the management of this case.

7. A 35-year-old female—lump breast. Investigation and treatment of a case of early carcinoma breast.

Vascular Disorders

8. A 40-year-old male admitted with gangrene of tips of the toes-management.

9. An individual reports to the OPD with a pulsatile mass in the abdomen with pain felt in the lumbar region and in the upper abdomen
   a. After clinical examination of the individual, how will you derive the diagnosis?
   b. What are the investigations you will do?
   c. How will you treat the disorder and if not treated what are the complications?

10. A 60-year-old male patient with history of claudication. Discuss the differential diagnosis, investigation and outline the management of this case.

GIT

11. A 70-year-old male with history of worsening constipation, bleeding per rectum and abdominal distension and pain. Discuss the differential diagnosis and management.

12. A 55-year-old male complains of bleeding per rectum on and off for one month, detail the various causes of the above condition and management of carcinoma rectum.

13. Discuss the differential diagnosis of hemetemesis and describe the treatment of portal cirrhosis.

14. Acute pancreatitis—etiology, pathophysiology, clinical features, complications and management.

15. Clinical picture of acute appendicitis. Management of acute............. in a 20-year-old male.

16. A young man with a history of two bouts of hemetemesis comes to the emergency service— possible causes(1), Investigations(4) Treatment of bleeding esophageal varices(4).

17. A 40-year-old male with hemetemesis and melena. Differential diagnosis and management of variceal bleed.

18. A 60-year-old patient has history of bleeding per rectum. Discuss the differential diagnosis, investigation and management of cancer of rectosigmoid region.

19. Essay: Classification of acute intestinal obstruction, clinical features, investigation and management of sigmoid volvulus.

20. Discuss the clinical features, differential diagnosis, investigation and complications of acute cholecystitis. Discuss the treatment of the individual and mention the recent trends.

21. Enumerate the complications of duodenal ulcer. How will you manage a case of perforation?

22. Discuss the etiology, pathology, investigation and treatment of ulcerative colitis.

23. Describe the etiology, clinical features, investigations and treatment of carcinoma stomach

24. Write about the clinical features, investigation and treatment of carcinoma head of pancreas.

25. What are the causes of obstructive jaundice. How do you investigate and manage a patient with obstructive jaundice?

26. A 45-year-old alcohol abuser for the past 10 years present with abdomen pain, weight loss, diabetes and steatorrhea since last week. Discuss briefly the DD and outline the principles of management.

Urology

27. A 20-year-old male came to the emergency department with sudden onset of pain in the flank radiating to the groin. His urine microscopic examination revealed hematuria. Discuss the differential diagnosis and management.

28. A 60-year-old male admitted with acute retention of urine. Discuss in detail the management with a special note on recent trends in the management of such patient. List the differential diagnosis.

29. Enumerate the causes of retention of urine. How will you manage a case of retention of urine in a 60-year-old man with enlarged prostate?

30. Causes of hematuria—investigation and treatment of traumatic hematuria.

31. A 40-year-old male—admitted with firm swelling of right scrotum—management.

32. Discuss etiology, pathology, clinical features and treatment carcinoma penis.

33. A 50-year-old male patient has come to the hospital with lump in the lumbar region. Discuss the causes, investigation and treatment of hypernephroma.

34. A 30-year-old male—testicular swelling—differential diagnosis(3)—investigations(3). How will you treat an early case of seminoma testis. Classify the tumors of the testis(3).

35. Discuss the causes of lower urinary obstruction. How do you manage a case of retention of urine in a 70-year-old man with BPH?

36. Discuss elaborately the causes, types, signs, symptoms and treatment of rupture of urinary bladder.

37. Write about the clinical features investigation and treatment of BPH.

38. A 60-year-old male patient complained of blood stained urine of recent onset. Write the possible causes, investigation that would be required in this patient to determine the cause and give an account on the principles of management.

39. A 30-year-old male patient with h/o hard testicular swelling. Write the differential diagnosis, investigation and outline the principles of management of testis tumor.

40. A 50-year-old patient comes to the hospital with hematuria
    a. Enumerate the possible causes.

b.   How will you investigate the case.
c.   Briefly outline the management of renal cell carcinoma.

Shock

41. What are the different types of shock. Discuss the pathophysiology, clinical features and management of hypovolemic shock.

Burns

42. A 60-year-old patient with near total burns sustained in a closed room. How will you evaluate this patient to assess the extent and the depth of burns? What are the other complications she can have due to the nature of the injury? Write about the evaluation and management of the case.

RTA

43. An individual is brought to the casualty with multiple injuries due to road traffic accident. Management of the individual at the hospital. Classification of fractures of the middle one-third of the face.

44. A 30-year-old male patient was brought to the accident and emergency department with the history of RTA. He was found to be unconscious. What are the possible causes? Write about the investigations and management.

45. A 10-year-old male patient with inability to open his mouth for the last 2 years. He has a history of fall from height about 3 years back. On examination, there is a scar under the chin and there is trismus. Discuss the management of this case.

46. A 45-year-old patient had been received unconscious, with history of motor vehicle accident 10 minutes back, with bleeding through oral and nasal cavities. What first aid would you provide this patient? How will you evaluate this patient to assess the severity of injury? Outline the management of this case.

Index

Page numbers followed by *f* refer to figure.